Ladies, Flat Booty?

Learn How to Grow glutes without growing legs and go from flat to plump in 30 days

http://amazon.com/review/create-review/asin= B09PD5JYJD

Written by MelloFit

Copyright _2021 - All rights reserved.

The content contained within this book may not be reproduced, duplicated, or transmitted without direct written permission from the author or the publisher.

Under no circumstances will any blame or legal responsibility be held against the publisher, or author, for any damages, reparation, or monetary loss due to the information contained within this book. Either directly or indirectly. You are responsible for your own choices, actions, and results.

Legal Notice:

This book is copyright protected. This book is only for personal use. You cannot amend, distribute, sell, use, quote or paraphrase any part, or the content within this book, without the consent of the author or publisher.

Disclaimer Notice:

Please note the information contained within this document is for educational and entertainment purposes only. All effort has been executed to present accurate, up to date, and reliable, complete information. No warranties of any kind are declared or implied. Readers acknowledge that the author is not engaging in the rendering of legal, financial, medical, or professional advice. The content within this book has been derived from various sources. Please consult a licensed professional before attempting any techniques outlined in this book.

By reading this document, the reader agrees that under no circumstances is the author responsible for any losses, direct or indirect, which are incurred as a result of the use of the information contained within this document, including, but not limited to, — errors, omissions, or inaccuracies.

Table of Contents

Table of Contents

INTRODUCTION

CHAPTER ONE

WHY YOUR BOOTY IS NOT GROWING AND WHAT TO DO ABOUT IT

CHAPTER 2

THE BUTT BROKEN DOWN INTO THREE MAJOR PARTS

CHAPTER THREE

BUILD THE BOOTY, NOT THE THIGHS

CHAPTER FIVE

A GLUTE PROGRAM THAT WILL PRODUCE THE BEST RESULTS

CHAPTER 6

EAT TO GROW YOUR BOOTY

CHAPTER 7

SHEDDING FAT WITHOUT LOSING GLUTE GAIN

CHAPTER 8

GLUTE STRETCHES

CONCLUSION

Just for You!

A gift to our readers.

Please enjoy your free copy of 7 myths regarding weight loss upon subscribing to join the MelloFit email list. Joining this email list will give you access to upcoming fitness content as well as an invitation to our fitness community on Facebook. This is a short document of the top 7 myths regarding weight loss and how to address them. The link for the email list is below.

https://mellofit.activehosted.com/f/1

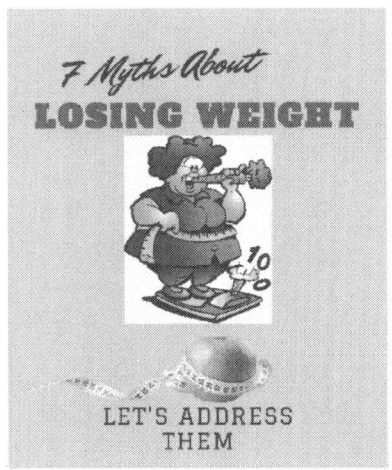

INTRODUCTION

Have you ever wished your butt would fill your jeans up and be firm or look like that of those models? Many girls dream of having butts that would make every head turn at every corner they take, and everywhere they pass. You want your butt to look sexy in everything you wear. While some women have it easy and naturally, some have to work their booty off (literally!) to get the booty of their dreams. Some go under the knife, while others want to achieve it through exercises. Perhaps, you have tried that method, and it seems like you are working your butt off, but you are not getting what you want. You end up with aching ties, and you are probably not able to walk properly for days, and you wonder what could be wrong.

Is it that you are doing the wrong exercises or doing the exercises the wrong way? It may seem like you may not get the booty you want even after all the pain you went through. If you are tired of your flat booty and would like to grow your booty in 30 days, you are reading the right book. This book will enlighten you on what you have been doing wrong, why you don't have the booty of your dreams, and how you can get it in 30 days.

In this book, you will get to know why you aren't growing your glutes the way you want and will provide a solution you can adopt to get it. You will discover if you have been doing the right exercise all along! This book will also help you understand your butt, the muscles, and the ones you need to target to get your desired results. Have you noticed that you have been growing your thighs instead of your butt? You might have been doing the wrong exercise, like squatting. If it's not squatting, what then should you do? This book will help you build your booty without growing your thighs.

Other things you will learn from reading this book are the SRA curve for our glute training, glute programs you can adopt to get the best results, the right diet for you to grow your butt, how you can shed your fat without losing your glute gains, and different glute stretches for your booty goals.

Are you ready to grow your booty in 30 days? Read, enjoy, and get the booty of your dreams.

CHAPTER ONE

WHY YOUR BOOTY IS NOT GROWING AND WHAT TO DO ABOUT IT

I know the drill: you wake up in the morning, put on your exercise gear, and you run for miles. Sometimes you skate, and sometimes, you ride a bicycle for a long time. Hoping with all the sweat you break; your booty would take some shape. I know how that feels; we've all been there. Doing the wrong things unknowingly and hoping to get the right results.

Many people think to get their dream body shape, they have to do many running, jogging, and other cardiovascular activities. They think breaking a sweat through steady-state cardio is how to build their glute muscles and get that well-rounded, bouncy booty that turns heads. In the real sense, this isn't the case at all. And if you've been relying on steady-state cardio to grow your booty, you've been doing the wrong thing. In this chapter, I will show you why steady-state cardio is the wrong approach to building your glute muscles and the right approach to take. Let's dive right in.

Why Steady State Cardio Is Not the Best for Growing Your Glute Muscles

Steady-state cardio is mostly the popular choice for many people who want to build their bodies. Why? It's a pretty straightforward approach and is mostly fun to do. It's easy to throw in your joggers and sneakers and go for a jog. You can even partner with a friend or neighbor while you chat along the way. You break some sweats, and then, that's it. It's quite a convenient route. So, why exactly is steady-state cardio not the right choice for you if you are trying to build the muscles in the right places? Especially when you are trying to grow your booty? Let's take a look.

Your body adjusts to Cardio

Steady-state cardio is tricky, mainly because of the way the body works. When you start with your cardiovascular exercise journey, you are likely to see quick, tremendous results. You are likely to lose a considerable number of pounds initially, and that tricks you to think your hard work is paying off. But after some time, your body stops losing weight, and it begins to store the fat it should be shedding.

So, let's say at the beginning of your exercises, your body burns about 300 calories for running 5 miles; after a while, your body begins to store in fat to increase its efficiency. So, instead of burning the regular 300 calories you used to burn, your start to burn 150 calories (hypothetically speaking). Why does this happen? When you run, jog, or do any cardiovascular activity, your body burns some fat. But over time, your body helps conserve this fat to produce more energy, so you can burn less fat, save your energy, and exercise for a more extended period.

Your body doesn't know you are trying to lose weight; rather, it thinks you are trying to perform a specific task. So, conversely, it works to help you build endurance over time by storing your fat for increased energy. This is why fitness experts suggest you adopt the muscle confusion approach, where you attempt different muscle exercises in your exercise routine, so your body doesn't adapt to the exercise you do. But this can be hard to keep up with too.

It requires more time

Steady-state cardio requires spending tons of time to get the tiniest result. For instance, you lose about 300 calories on a 5 miles exercise at the beginning of the exercise, and over time you burn 150 miles for the same 5 miles exercise, then you have to run further than 5 miles to burn the initial 300 calories. It's more like you are going back and forth. And you'd be spending more time and more effort to get a little result. One more thing: your body increases its efficiency as you go. So, you will keep running longer to lose the calories you have in mind. Thereby taking your time and sweats for little outcome. You should spend those time doing something that works to bring the results you need.

It puts you at risks of Injuries

Steady-state cardio exercises have limited variations, so you may get stuck on an exercise rut. This means you would have to repeat the same kind of exercises, and apart from the fact that your body will get used to these exercises, you also run at risk of injuries.

Steady-state Cardio Misconceptions

Cardio-vascular activities come with their misconceptions. And it's probably these misconceptions that make many people think they can build their body muscle and shape with steady-state cardio activities. You are probably familiar with seeing people jog and run on your street. Most times, these early-morning runners are usually your body goals: with a well-fit and well-shaped body you want. And somehow, you think they got this body from jogging every morning, but the truth is, it doesn't always work that way.

Many people run, jog and perform other cardiovascular activities because they are fit for them. It's possible the person who jogs every morning in your neighborhood already had that shape before she even started her running or jogging routine. Just like other athletic activities, people run, jog, play basketball because they already have the body for it. And not because they hope to have the body through these exercises.

Why squats won't grow your booty

Ever asked anyone how to grow your booty? Do squats, they will say. But then you do squats for months, and your booty doesn't grow one bit. Ever wondered why? The reason is simple. Squats don't target your glutes specifically, so they aren't enough to grow your glutes muscles. Your glutes muscles are located at the lowest part of the squat position, so it's only when you squat the right way that you can hit your glutes muscles just a little.

Your legs, thighs, and hamstrings do the major work when you perform squats. This is why you feel pains at your thigh region when you squat rather than the butt you are targeting. With squats, you see great improvements in your thigh region, but you only get to see the tiniest improvement on your butt even when you squat the right way.

The Real Way to Grow Your Booty

Lifting weight is the real way to get the booty of your dreams. It is more than an efficient medicine because it brings tremendous results when done correctly. They are effective because they help you skyrocket your metabolism and metabolic rate to shed excess fat and build your body muscle in the right places. Does lifting weight sound a bit off the radar for you? Why though?

Here's Why You Aren't Lifting - Weight

Let's check out the possible reasons you haven't hit the gym to lift those weight yet:

You are afraid you will get all buffed off

This is one of the hottest discussions that never gets old. Many ladies are afraid of weightlifting because they want to tone their bodies without getting bulk up. Here's the thing: the idea of getting bulk up as a lady is a misconception (or would I rather call it a myth?) on its own. We aren't structured as men, so we can't get all buffed up when we lift a weight. We don't have the same testosterone level as men (men have 16 times higher testosterone levels), so there's no way we will get bulk up when we lift a weight.

It's essential to lift weight to gain a build your body muscles to get that perfect booty you want. However, you can't tone a specific part of your body only. It's impossible to lose weight in just one part of your body because our bodies don't work that way. We have to lose fat from every aspect of our body. This is why lifting muscle is essential if you are looking to lose weight in some part of your body, and it even works better to define those muscles and direct them to the places you want them to be.

You don't want to get injured

You probably don't want to hit the gym because you are afraid you will get hurt when you lift a weight. All that weight-lifting equipment can look scary, and it's probably the reason you haven't hit the gym yet. The truth is: you can't get hurt, when necessary, precautions are taken. Besides, there would always be expert gym trainers to guide you as you lift a weight. They know the right weight to give you, and they won't give you more than you can handle. But you can't keep letting fear grip you down from doing the things you want to do. So, get your butt in the gym and do some weightlifting!

You aren't confident enough

Maybe you haven't hit the gym because you are not confident enough. You probably think you can't do it, or you think you don't have enough strength and capacity to do so, especially if you consider it a manly activity. It's normal to feel that way when you haven't made any attempt at weightlifting before. However, the first step to overcome your lack of confidence is to try. If you don't try, you will never know how much you can do. But if you, you will be surprised at how far you can go, and this realization will give you the confidence you need to continue. So never lose focus on the big goal, and do not let your fear and insecurities stop you from getting what you want.

Here's Why You Should Start Weightlifting

Now, let's talk about the benefits of weightlifting. Why exactly should you get over your fear and hit the gym to lift some weight?

Lose Weight Better

Contrary to popular opinion, you tend to lose weight better through weightlifting than steady-state cardio. Many people don't lift to get bulk up; they lift weight to shed fat and stay fit. Here is how it works: your body has a massive ability to burn fat when you exercise and after you exercise. More so, after lifting weight, your body takes in extra oxygen hours and days after. This activity is referred to as EPOC (Excess post-exercise oxygen consumption). When this happens, your metabolic rate increases, and you shed fat better.

Burn fat more, gain muscle better

Weightlifting increases your strength and lean muscle mass, which helps you burn calories better. You experience more muscle contractions, which enable you to burn extra calories. An increased lean muscle mass also means more muscle contractions to burn fat more.

Get your perfect body

Weightlifting helps you build your muscle, and when this happens, your body begins to take the perfect hourglass shape you love. You become curvier, and your booty grows bigger. This is because weightlifting helps you lose weight, but the weight come in muscle tissue.

Improve your bone Health

As you grow other, the chances of losing your bone and muscle mass become high. More so, because postmenopausal women no longer secrete estrogen, they are at higher chances of osteoporosis. But weightlifting helps prevent loss of bone mass, thereby preventing decreasing the chances of osteoporosis.

Why Should You Choose Weightlifting over Steady-state Cardio?

There are many reasons to opt for weightlifting instead of steady-state cardio, here are more reasons to choose weightlifting over steady-state cardio:

1. Weight-lifting sessions are less time-consuming than steady-state cardio.

2. They are effective, exciting, and challenging. You have a sense of fulfillment after every work-out session.

3. Weightlifting helps you burn more calories faster. Weightlifting involves burning calories during and after the weight-lifting sessions. Research reveals instead of glycogen, your body burns fat as fuel after 24 hours of every weight-lifting session.

Weightlifting is by far a better alternative to steady-state cardio. With consistent effort, you are bound to see results in no time.

Your Glute Muscles Need to be Strength Trained

When trying to grow a nice, curvy booty, you should know this: the muscles are deeply involved. And as such, you have to train them effectively to achieve the type of booty you want. The shape of your butt is defined by muscles called glutes (gluteus maximus, gluteus medius, and gluteus minimus).

Although steady-state cardio exercises such as running, hiking, and climbing can do something for your glute's muscles, they can only do a little. To achieve glaring progress with your butt's size, you need to be able to train them specifically. When you train the muscles in your butt specifically, you can reach hypertrophy- the growth in the size of your muscles.

The idea is pretty straightforward- if you want to grow your triceps, you focus on your triceps and not your biceps. So, if you're going to train your glutes, why focus on your legs? Strength training helps you hit your glutes muscles directly to achieve a firmer and more rounded butt. They put enough pressure on your glutes so you can achieve hypertrophy on your glutes in no time.

Smart Strategies to Grow Your Glute Muscles

Below are the top strategies to adopt to grow your glute muscles the right way:

Perform exercises that target your glute muscles

Growing your glutes muscles means you have to do away with generic exercises and target exercises that really focus on your glute muscles. Exercises targeted at the glute muscle area will enable you to see quick results with your butt. There are different examples of exercises you can explore, more on later in this chapter.

Practice the progressive overload

Adopting the progressive overload technique facilitates your glutes muscles' growth. Progressive overload is a straight training theory that involves continuously increasing the amount of resistance your muscles are used to.

This means you will keep adding to the weight you work with over time to challenge your muscle for better results with your glutes.

The women who have the biggest perfect booties with straight training exercises challenge themselves using the progressive overload technique.

Master the rule of thirds

Practicing the rule of thirds helps bring excellent outcomes with your glute muscles' growth. When training your glute muscles, the rule of third means one-third of the glute exercises should be horizontal, one-third should be vertical, and one-third should be lateral. This is also applicable to the effort and weight you put in when training your glute muscles. For lower reps: one-third of the weight can be heavy; for medium reps, one-third of the weight should be medium; for higher reps, one-third of the weight should be light. The rule of thirds ensures you achieve the best balance when exercising your glutes.

Maintain healthy nutrition

Your work-out sessions at the gym and your lifestyle work hand-in-hand to give you the perfect booty you want. It doesn't matter how hard you work at the gym; if you under eat or do not maintain a nutritious diet that complements your work-out sessions, your glute muscles won't grow to reach their best potentials. When targeting the growth of your glute muscles, it would help to increase your diet. This is because strength training helps you burn fat and grow your muscles at the same time. So, if you eat healthily and at a considerable amount, you are bound to see results faster. But don't just focus on the quantity of what you eat; ensure to keep your meals highly nutritious too.

Weightlifting is the best route to take if you want to grow your booty in the best way possible. While it isn't always easy, it sure is the way to go for real results in a reasonable amount of time. Plus, it doesn't only help grow your butt; it also comes with numerous health benefits, some of which have been discussed in this chapter.

CHAPTER 2

THE GLUTES BROKEN DOWN INTO THREE MAJOR PARTS

Glutes, butts, gluteal, buttocks, gluteus, backside, derriere, rump, tush, keister, caboose, booty, nates, fanny. The list is long. Glutes are the strongest and largest muscles in your body. Glutes have so many different names for that one part of the body which almost everyone intends to tone, tighten and build. The most energetic and most extensive group of muscles in the human body is the gluteal, consisting of the gluteus medius, gluteus maximus, and gluteus minimus. Apart from the three significant parts earlier mentioned, the gluteal muscles also include the hamstrings, consisting of semitendinosus, semimembranosus, and biceps femoris. These groups of muscles function together to rotate, extend and abduct the hip. They also help to stabilize the pelvis, especially during running, climbing, and running.

Furthermore, glutes are another name for the three major parts of the gluteal muscles that form the pelvis and then insert into the femur. For example, the three major parts of the gluteal, commonly referred to as buttocks, are as follows:

- The gluteus minimus
- Gluteus medius
- Gluteus maximus

The name gluteus has its origin from the Latin version of the Greek word *gloutos*, which means buttock. It is important to note that the gluteal muscles do other things in your body apart from just hanging out on your back. So, if you're the type that takes pleasure engaging in exercises such as running, walking, rotating your hip joints, or jumping, then it's high time you thanked your glutes.

The gluteal part of the human body is an anatomical region located behind the pelvic girdle close to the center end of the femur. The muscles in this area, however, place the lower limb at the hip joint on motion. Meanwhile, the muscles of the gluteal region can be divided into two different groups, which include deep lateral rotators and superficial abductors and extenders.

Deep Lateral Rotators

The deep lateral rotators consist of smaller muscles that react majorly to rotate the femur laterally. These muscles include the piriformis, gemellus inferior, quadratus femoris, obturator internus and gemellus superior.

Superficial Abductors and Extenders

The superficial abductors and extenders comprise large muscles that extend and abduct the femur. They include the gluteus minimus, gluteus medius, tensor fascia lata and gluteus maximus.

The arterial supply to these muscles happens through the internal iliac artery's inferior and superior artery branches, after which venous drainage follows the arterial supply.

Read further to know more about the groups of gluteal muscles, innervations, attachments, and actions. We shall also consider the clinical relevance of muscle disorder and the benefits you'll derive from training your gluteal muscles.

The Superficial Muscles

The superficial muscles in the gluteal region are comprised of the tensor fascia lata and the three glutei. The superficial muscles mainly perform the act of abducting and extending the lower limb at the hip joint.

Gluteus Maximus

The gluteus maximus is the main gluteal muscles. Just as its name, Maximus, appears, it is the biggest and most muscular among all the gluteal muscles. Another way to describe the gluteus maximus is that it is one of the strongest muscles in the human body. It also appears to be the most superficial, thus, producing the shape of the bottom. It plays a lead role in abducting and laterally rotating the hips, and it also assists in hip extension, which pulls the leg backward.

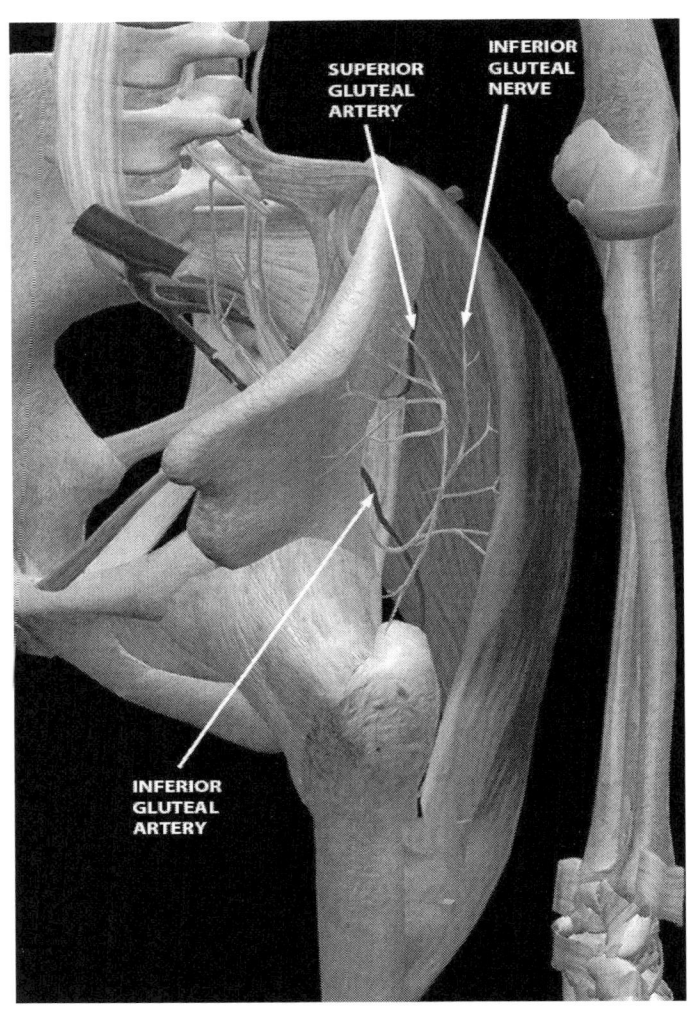

Visiblebody.com

- *Actions*

This is the primary extensor of the thigh. Its function is to help with lateral rotation. As a matter of fact, it is only applied when a force like climbing or running is required.

- *Blood supply*

Inferior and superior gluteal arteries

- *Innervation*

Innervation is the inferior gluteal nerve.

- *Attachments*

Attachments stem from the posterior (gluteal) surface of the coccyx, sacrum, and ilium. It slides across the bottom at a forty-five-degree angle and then inserts into the femur's gluteal tuberosity and iliotibial tract.

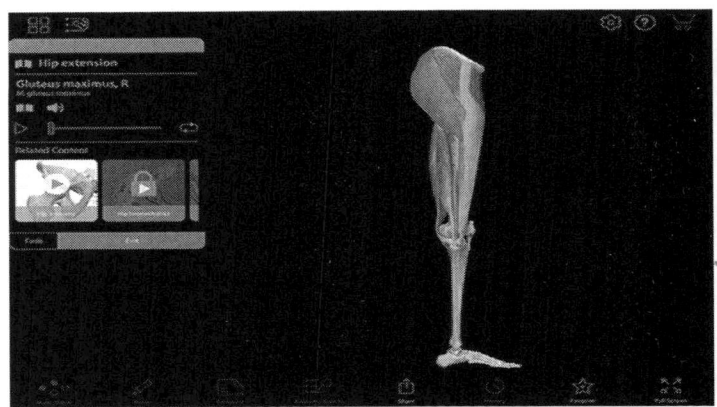

Gluteus Medius

As a matter of fact, the gluteus medius muscle is obviously the middle-sized gluteal muscle. Its shape is like that of a fan, and it lies between the gluteus minimus and the gluteus maximus. Therefore, it has almost the same shape as the gluteus minimus, and they function the same way too.

It is a significant mover in medial rotation, lateral rotation, and hip abduction. It also helps maintain the pelvis's side-to-side stability, enabling the gluteus minimus to keep the pelvis aligned adequately during motion and single-leg balancing.

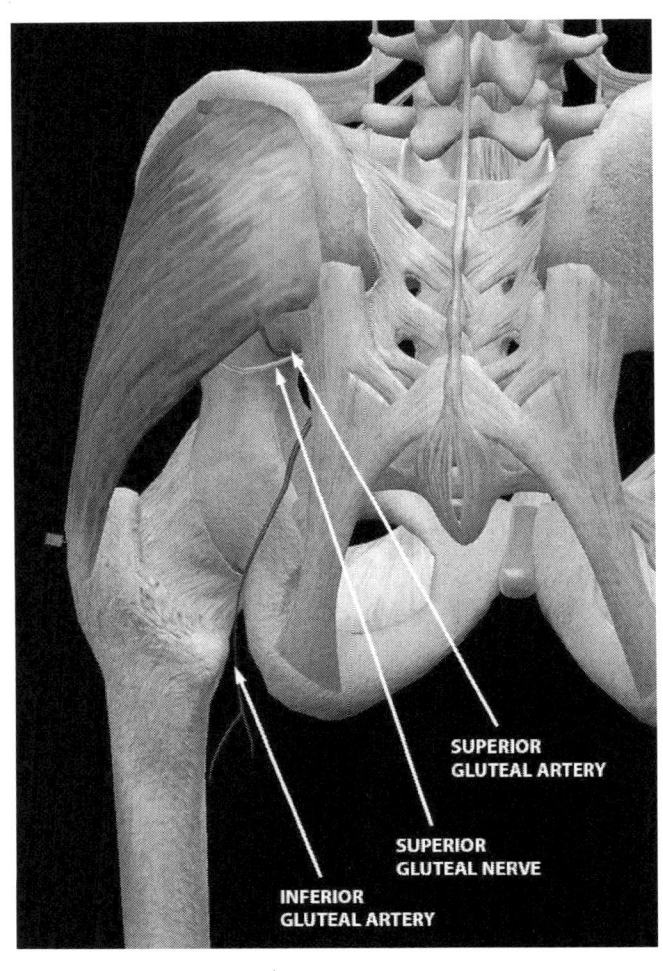

Visiblebody.com

- *Innervation*

The innervation of the gluteus medius is the superior gluteal nerve.

- *Actions*

Gluteus medius captures and medially rotates the lower limb. During movement, it safeguards the pelvis, avoiding the pelvic drop of the opposite limb. Meanwhile, the posterior fibers of the gluteus medius are also perceived to produce a tiny amount of side rotation.

- *Blood supply*

Inferior and superior gluteal arteries

- *Attachments*

This has its root from the gluteal surface of the ilium and encloses into the lateral surface of the superior trochanter.

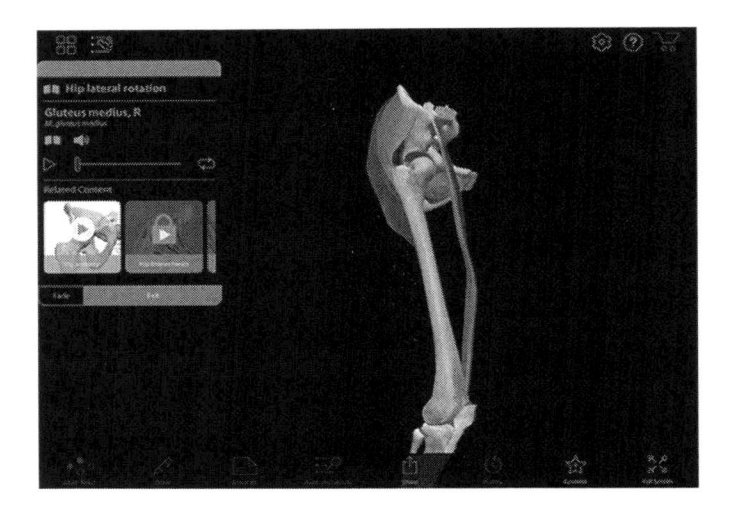

Visiblebody.com

Gluteus Minimus

The gluteus minimus is the lightest and most profound of the superficial gluteal muscles. Its function is to capture the thigh and ensure the pelvis and hips fit during exercises such as running, standing on one leg, or walking. Apart from providing maximum fitness for the hips and pelvis, its anterior portion offers internal rotation for the thigh, whereas its posterior part offers external rotation. It is, however, essential to note that gluteus minimus does not appear immense, and it works on the gluteus medius.

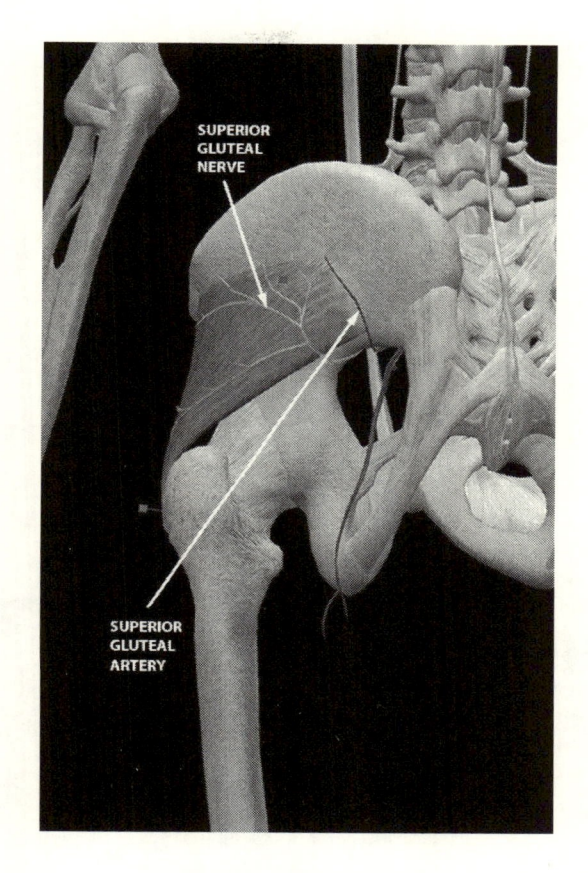

Visiblebody.com

- ***Actions***

It seizes and medially alternates the lower limb. During motion, it fortifies the pelvis, stopping the pelvic drop of the contradictory stem.

- **Attachments**

It has its origin from the ilium and unites to create a tendon, thereby implanting to the frontal side of the greater trochanter.

- **Innervation**

Gluteus minimus has a higher gluteal nerve.

- **Blood supply**

Superior gluteal artery

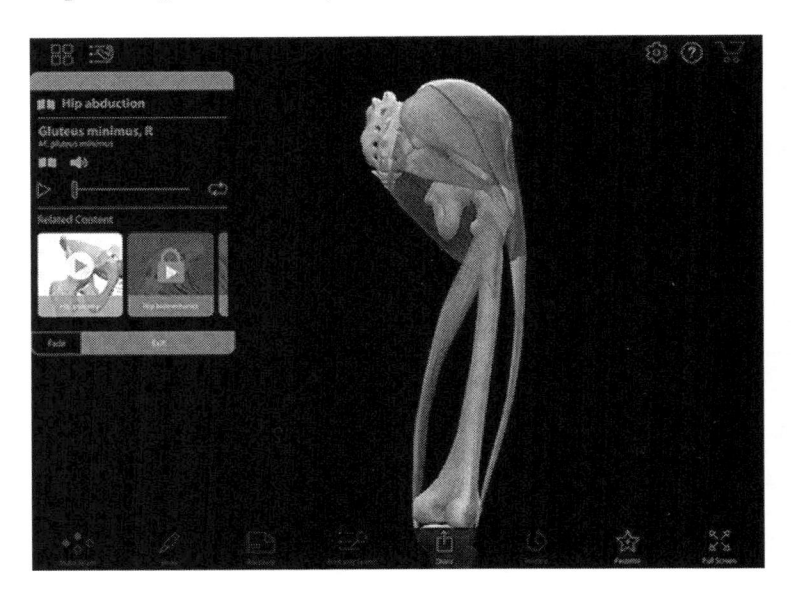

Visiblebody.com

Tensor Fascia Lata

Tensor fascia lata is a minute superficial muscle found around the iliac crest's anterior axis. Its function is to tighten the fascia lata and abduct and medially rotate the limb on the lower region.

- *Attachments*

It has its origin from the anterior iliac crest and attaches to the anterior superficial iliac spine (ASIS). It inserts into the iliotibial tract, which connects itself to the adjacent condyle of the tibia.

- *Innervation*

Tensor fascia lata's innervation is the superficial gluteal nerve.

- *Actions*

It helps the gluteus minimus and gluteus medius to abduct and medially rotate the lower limb. It also gives support to the gait cycle.

Clinical Relevance: Damage to the Superior Gluteal Nerve

The superior gluteal nerve stimulates the gluteus minimus and gluteus medius. These muscles play critical roles in innervating the pelvis during movement. While in the standing position, the gluteus medius and minimus contract when you raise the contralateral leg, which prevents the pelvis from dropping on that side. If the superior gluteal nerve gets damaged, the previously described muscles become paralyzed, making it unsteady along the way. Meanwhile, a characteristic finding of gluteal muscle weakness is referred to as *the Trendelenburg sign*.

As a matter of fact, the patient produces the Trendelenburg sign when they are asked to stand on each leg without any assistance. Again, a pelvic drop will occur on the unsupported, and this time, more positively. You will be able to recognize a pelvic sign by paying attention to the level of the iliac crests on the two sides of the legs. An excellent example of this is if the gluteal muscles become weak, the right side of the pelvis will drop immediately; the patient stands on their left leg, while the right leg doesn't have any support.

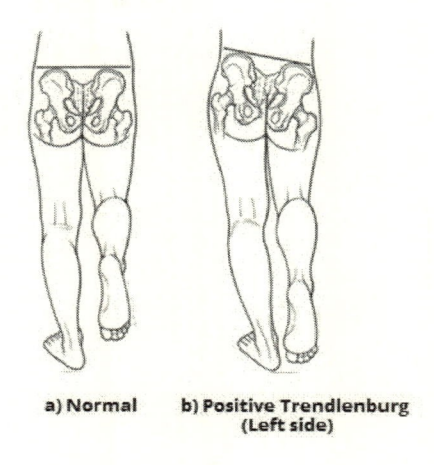

a) Normal   b) Positive Trendlenburg
(Left side)

Teachmeanatomy.info

The Deep Muscles

The deep muscles are a set of smaller muscles found beneath the gluteus minimus. The primary functions of these muscles are to rotate the lower limb laterally. They also stabilize the hip joint by pulling the femoral head into the acetabulum of the pelvis.

The Piriformis

The piriformis muscle is a primary landmark in the gluteal area of the body. It is the most superficial of the deep muscles.

- *Attachments*

It stems from the anterior surface of the sacrum. After which, it moves inferno-laterally through the greater sciatic foramen to insert into the greater trochanter of the thigh bone.

- *Actions*

The piriformis muscle functions as lateral rotation and abduction.

- *Innervation*

Nerve to the piriformis.

Obturator Internus

The obturator internus is the formation of the lateral walls of the pelvic cavity. The Gemelli muscles and the obturator internus are often seen as one muscle, known as the triceps coxae.

- *Attachments*

It has its origin from the ischium and the pubis found at the obturator foramen. It moves through the lesser sciatic foramen and is attached to the more prominent trochanter of the femur.

- *Innervation*

Nerve to obturator internus

- *Actions*

Lateral abduction and rotation.

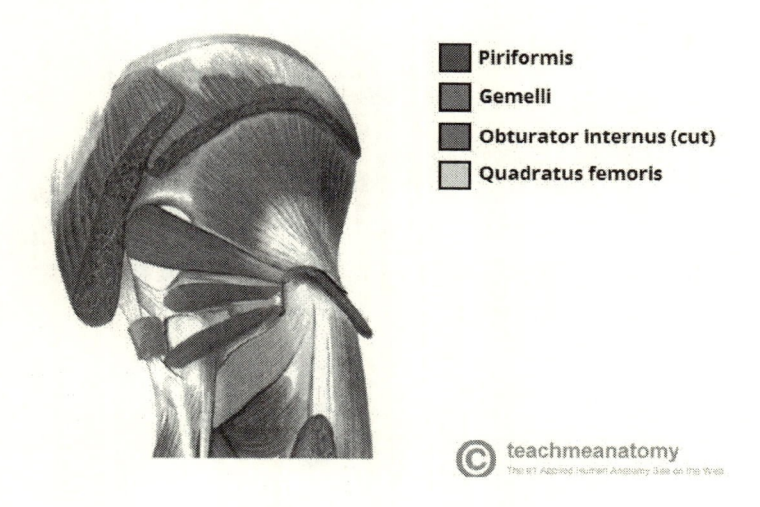

Teachmeanatomy.info

The Gemelli: Inferior and Superior

The Gemelli, which includes the superior and interior, are two triangular and narrow muscles. They stand apart through the help of the obturator internus tendon.

- *Attachments*

The inferior gemellus muscle originates from the ischial tuberosity, while the superior from the ischial spine. The two gemellus muscles attach to the more prominent trochanter of the thigh bone.

- *Innervation*

The inferior gemellus muscle is innervated by the nerve to quadratus femoris, while the superior gemellus is innervated by the nerve to obturator internus.

- *Actions*

Lateral rotation and abduction.

Quadratus Femoris

The quadratus femoris is a flat and square-shaped muscle. It is located underneath the Gemelli and obturator internus. Among all the deep gluteal muscles, the quadratus femoris happens to be the most inferior.

- *Actions*

Lateral rotation

- *Attachments*

It stems from the lateral side of the ischial tuberosity and glues to the quadrate tuberosity on the intertrochanteric crest.

- *Innervation*

Nerve to quadratus femoris

Clinical Relevance: Landmark of the Gluteal Region

One cannot overemphasize the presence of piriformis in the gluteal region. It represents an anatomical landmark in the glutei. As the muscle moves via the greater sciatic foramen, it separates the gluteal region into a superior and an inferior part. This process speaks volumes of the nerves and vessels that supply the region. It is pertinent to note that the ideal gluteal vessels and nerves develop into the gluteal area in a way superior to the piriformis and work the other way round for the inferior gluteal nerve.

More so, one can use piriformis to figure out the sciatic nerve. Then, the sciatic nerve runs into the gluteal area, visible as a flat band, directly inferior to the piriformis and approximately two centimeters wide.

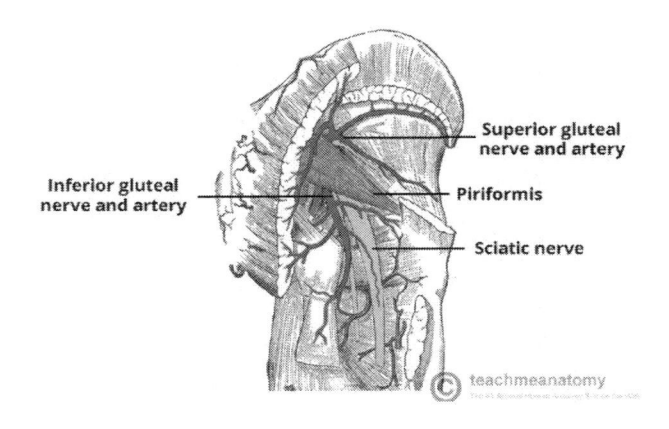

Teachmeanatomy.info

Other Facts You Should Know About Glute

Here are some facts and findings of glute:

Hormone Influences Distribution of Fat

Every individual has a layer of fat that mitigates the growth of their gluteal parts. As a matter of fact, sitting for long in a position seems uncomfortable. However, the amount of fat that people have is inclined by their sex hormones. It is worth noting that estrogen spurs up biologically female individuals to gather fat on their buttocks and thighs.

You'll Be Less Prone to Certain Injuries.

The truth is, if you have strong gluteal muscles, be sure that muscles will contribute to pelvic stability, posture, and improved balance. In addition, with a strong core, the improved pelvic stability approved by the glutes will go a long way to minimize the danger of a range of sports-related lower-body injuries, including shin splints and the runner's knee.

Howbeit, there is diverse aerobics you can engage in that will help strengthen the glutes. Few among these many exercises include:

- Leg lifts
- Bridges
- Lunges
- Squats

Unregulated Control of The Gluteal Muscles Can Cause Gluteal Pain

If you do not take proper care of your gluteal muscles, you may end up sustaining an injury or chronic pain in your butt. Overusing and insufficient control of the gluteal muscles can result in gluteal tendinopathy. Gluteal tendinopathy happens when pain springs up from the upper leg and the gluteal region. It is usually caused by the decline of the tendons on there. Unnecessary activity or inactivity might cause the condition to spring up.

As time unfolds, the ligaments of the gluteal muscles, primarily the gluteus medius and gluteus minimus, can experience what is known as microtears, thus, leading to gluteal tendinopathy, which implies tendon pain.

Gluteal tendinopathy is sometimes caused by improper control of the hip and gluteal muscles, which exerts so much stress on the tendons. For instance, tedious overworking can lead to tendinosis, which is a gradual deterioration of collagen fibers in the tendons.

Frequently, gluteal tendinopathy occurs together with trochanteric bursitis, that is, inflammation of one of the fluid-filled sacs found around the hip joint to cause more Trochanteric Pain Syndrome, pain on the bottom and outside of the hips.

How To Grow Stronger Butt Muscles?

Anyone who wants to train for strong glutes should have had her 'whys' spelled out. I need to let you know that the booty kickbacks and band walks you do every week isn't going to give you your long-awaited result. At least, not them alone. The truth is you need to train every part of your gluteal complex. What this means is, you'll need to train for hip abduction, single leg balance, stability, and hip extension. You may be wondering why lifestyle modification alone isn't sufficient to make you have that round and perky butt you've always dreamed of having. It would be best if you did this because your glutes are made up of both slow-twitch fibers; that is why you should train them in a mix of both high and low ranges, isometric holds, and slow and fast tempos. If your goal is to build rounder or bigger glutes, and you see no big deal in spending time growing the muscles, then there is every tendency that you'll be able to change the shape of your butts.

In a general sense, the gluteus maximus is the amalgamation of fast-twitch muscle fibers. Rapid-firing fibers are selected for bursts of power or speed, and slow-twitch muscle fibers are the workhorses during aerobic exercises. However, some research shows that the gluteus minimum and medius primarily contain slow-twitch muscles. The implication of this is that the butt muscles can profit from both strength training with low reps and high load, like heavy-weight squats, to work the fast-twitch muscles, and with high reps, download and endurance exercises like climbing of stairs, that is, working slow-twitch muscles, and running. That aside, a cluster of non-squat strength moves essential key for building stronger glutes, and it isn't a bad idea to include glute activation exercises at the start of your workouts. This will help ensure that all your muscles are firing.

As a matter of fact, a big part of your buttock's experience is often dictated by the layer of fat that covers the said glutes, which is that part that you twerk with. A considerable amount of the female posterior is fat, while the exact muscles are shaped like men. However, there's a slight difference in orientation simply because the pelvis is a bit wider. However, if you aim to lose fat in a bid to pursue rounder and firmer glutes, then be sure that you'll need to follow a healthy calorie-appropriate diet and add regular HIT or cardio on most days to reduce fat all over. Doing so will help you determine your calorie intake.

And if you want to grow muscles, you'll also need to be mindful of your calorie intake and strength training exercises accordingly. Always have it at the back of your mind that if you're dead set on using exercise and diet to modify the ability and appearance of your butt, be sure that you're working towards achieving the best glutes muscles for your body. This is something anyone who wants to grow her butt and move it should know that it is possible, as long as you can put your mind to attaining it.

Benefits of Building the Glutes Muscles

Did you know that you tend to have fewer injuries when you have strong glute muscles, perform better, and most of all grow a nice butt? Gluteus, Gluteus, and Gluteus maximus are the three muscles that work together to stabilize the pelvis and maintain proper movement in the hips. The absence of this group of muscles in the human body will not make you actively engage in activities including squatting, rotating, twerking, twisting, or spending so much time on anything as long as it concerns the lower body. This is because any person who doesn't make out time to grow her glutes will find it difficult moving the lower body. So, working more on the strength of your glutes can help increase mobility, flexibility and generally make the day such as stair climbing, sitting, running, lifting heavy weights, and more activities easier.

The truth is, a well-trained butt isn't just lovely to behold; but has several other benefits like alleviating your lower hip, back, and knee pain, improving your posture, reducing bone density loss, eliminating stubborn abdominal pooch, and enhancing athletic performance. Why is this so? Because muscles burn more calories at rest than fat does, as such, increasing lean muscles through glutes training can fast-track fat loss and also help to keep it off.

There are, however, few ways that were growing your glutes can improve your overall performance. Among which are:

Improved posture

Many people suffer from poor postures because of sitting disease. However, building your glutes muscles will provide you with an improved posture. This is because weak, shortened hip flexors, tight, over-stretched hip extensors, and glutes that do not remember how to activate all contribute to the most commonly observed postural deviations, such as kyphosis-lordosis and swayback. Working on your glutes will make you push your abdomen out, having the mindset of a butt even in the absence of excess belly fat.

Another thing you can do to help improve your posture is by including lunges, deadlifts, and squats in your strength training exercise. Meanwhile, you should stretch out the opposing hip flexors to better posture and reduce fat belly. This is one of the easiest and quickest ways to lose more pounds and be about two inches taller.

Reduces pain and prevents injury

Healthy glutes provide the utmost support for the lower back. When the glutes aren't fit enough to perform their hip extension function, the muscles that weren't made for the job will take over. These muscles may sometimes become overstressed, amounting to compression and pain in the hips, lumbar spine, and knees. Because the glutes are also hip stabilizers, weak gluteus can make the whole body not correctly align, exposing you to injuries such as shin splints, tears, and iliotibial (IT) band syndrome, anterior cruciate ligament (ACL), and Achilles tendonitis. To protect your ankles, knees, and hips, it would be best to strengthen your gluteal muscles with single-leg deadlifts, weighted clamshells, and hip thrusts.

Fat loss and maintenance

Engaging in gluteal muscle exercises will make you shed fat and also help maintain your physique. Fat loss requires a daily caloric discrepancy. So, you should burn more calories than the one you consume, and you'll be amazed about how much fat you've lost. On the contrary, with adipose tissue, muscle is metabolically active, which implies that your muscles will burn calories from stored fat even when you aren't engaging in exercises. To buttress this, some studies show that for every pound of muscle you build, your body will burn up to fifty calories per day. This is possible because glutes and hamstrings are two of the largest groups of muscles in the body as such their one cannot underestimate their contribution to fat loss.

To achieve this, try integrating several lunges and squats in a whole-body compound lift style circuit to torch fat, build muscles, and continue burning calories for a day or two after you're done working out.

You will feel better.

Since the gluteal muscles are the largest in the human body, if they are strong and engage in physical exercises every week, be sure that cardiovascular exercises and upper body workouts will not be challenging to do. You will feel better running or walking up the stairs, and you'll equally observe a difference in your daily movement.

Your bone density will improve.

Bone density increases between five and ten years after humans reach skeletal maturity.

Starting from the age of thirty, the old and damaged bone is resorbed faster than new bone is formed, leading to an increased risk of contracting osteoporosis, a condition where one has a progressive bone disease, and osteopenia, that is, a state where one experiences lower than the average bone density.

Engaging in exercises that make the bones undergo mechanical stress, such as running, lower bodyweight training, and some forms of yoga, can help you delay and even converse the effects of age-related bone-density loss. If you want fast results, it would be best for you to incorporate them into your training.

Strong glutes are good for esthetics.

This is one of the key reasons that people start their glutes training journey. Although, it may not be the most important reason. However, it is a reasonable goal to have, and if chasing a beautiful perky butt will make you feel good about yourself, then it's not bad if you go for it.

Increased athletic performance

The gluteus maximus can generate a massive amount of power. This enormous power is capable of translating into acceleration, endurance, vertical distance, and sports-specific speed. Working on the hips to powerfully extend and thrust the body forwards will help give your body the ability to jump, cycle, and run faster, longer, and more complicated.

To get maximum results, try to train your lower body a day or two, especially when you're not scheduled for a cycle or a long run. Don't forget to stretch and foam roll as you go on to maintain hip flexibility and mobility.

Studies have shown that athletes who focus more on developing power and strength in their hips, posterior chains, and glutes tend to perform better than those who neglect this training.

Easy Glute Exercises

Below are some of the glute exercises you can incorporate into your weekly leg routine:

Bridges

- Lay on the floor with your back
- Set a machine ball at your feet
- Bridge your pelvis up and down
- Squeeze your butt at the top.

You can try this glute exercise up to three times of twelve to fifteen reps.

Lunges

- Position yourself (barbell) on your shoulders/back
- Lunge up to fifteen times on each side
- Go as low as you can, but ensure not to touch the ground
- Make sure each knee doesn't go behind the other

You can try three sets of thirty lunges, ensuring to alternate your legs, fifteen times, each.

Kettlebell swings

- Position yourself, squatting
- Hold a 20-20lb kettlebell between your legs
- Thrust the kettlebell forward as you stand up
- Lower the kettlebell between your legs again as you squat back down.

You can try three sets of kettlebell swings about fifteen to twenty times.

Glute Training Mistakes You Should Avoid

Now that you know about the significant factors in solid glutes and you actively engage in them yet, your butt isn't protruding as you expect. You may likely be doing it the wrong way, hence, getting little or no results at all. It's sad to let you know that this is a common mistake people train their glute muscles to make, and over time, it keeps extending from the lower back to the hip, leaving them with no clue of what to do.

To avoid this common mistake, make it a great deal to engage your core, let your chin down, and tuck in your pelvis. Although you may not be able to extend your hips as high as you should, this action will help you feel the exercises in your glutes.

That aside, the leading cause of this issue could also be a weak core. Your inability to engage your body may lead to the trunk's instability, which may likely amount to you finding it difficult to activate your glutes.

In a nutshell, your glutes are vital. The above reasons prove to you that if you want to maintain better posture, improve your balance, explore your body, and enjoy a host of many other benefits, you need to be at the forefront, training your gluteal muscles.

CHAPTER THREE
BUILD THE BOOTY, NOT THE THIGHS

We all understand that squats are great. But can squats get you that strongly desired glute size? Now, unless you are genetically blessed in the glute region, then squats alone would probably not do the trick.

And with the increase in the number of people who crave a great and well-defined exterior, it has suddenly become everyone's fitness goal to build their glute. Besides, having a great and strong glute isn't a bad fitness goal. A strong glute has a whole host of fitness and physical benefits.

It is understandable trainers and researchers are working tirelessly on ways to effective ways to build bigger, stronger glutes and that more women are attempting to gain weight through food and exercise.

It makes sense that most trainers and researchers have been working on pinpointing the most efficient ways to which people can get bigger, stronger glutes and, of course, more women are trying to gain weight through diet and exercise

While squats can and should be a component of any lower-body workout, they aren't the optimal move for glute development. They would not only increase the size of your glute, but they would also end up increasing your thighs too.

Here are ways to go about getting stronger, greater glutes that go beyond the staple movement.

Why do squats not target the glutes specifically?

Squats are an important workout with several health advantages. Squats can help you lose weight and body fat, making your buttocks and thighs appear smaller, tighter, more toned, and compact.

This is because squats are a great way to build muscle, which is a great way to reduce body fat. Over time the body would experience a lean out, there would be more muscles than fat, there would be a change in body composition, making your metabolism faster, resulting in a change in shape. Then the thighs would be toned, the glutes lifted and become firmer, and they appear shapelier. And because muscles take up less room than fat, it means that while you may be building muscles and shape in a particular r area, it would still become smaller.

If you're very skinny or have very little body fat, though, you can produce around, shapely butt by strengthening your thigh and glute muscles with lower-body strength training. So, if you're wondering if you can "develop a booty" if you weren't born with one, the answer is a yes. However, the extent would be determined by the routine you choose, your level of dedication and intensity, and the added effect from dead weight too.

Squats primarily target your glutes and thighs (hamstrings and quadriceps), but they also target your core, oblique muscles, lower back, calves, and ankle complex. It can be a total body workout depending on the weight you're using, how you're holding it, and the squat variant you're doing.

However, while squat works on your glutes, it works on the thighs and abs, which won't make it an ideal routine workout for people who want to only improve on their posterior and glute muscles. Focusing on any form of squat would give you your desired result, but with added dead weight in places you wouldn't want, the best advice is to grow your glute using glute isolation exercise as the squat isn't idle for just your glutes only.

Growing Your Glutes and Not Your Thighs

The gluteal muscles are those muscles that make up the buttocks. The human body contains very few muscle groups that are as significant to the glutes.

Because they are placed in the central part of the body, the glutes are necessary for lower-body movement and upper-body support.

Strength in the glutes is required for almost every exercise that involves your legs, thighs, or hips. There are very few workouts that entirely isolate the glutes, which is a vital muscle group for body mobility. However, there are a variety of effective glute exercises that primarily stimulate the glutes while also reducing the activity of adjacent muscles, allowing the glutes to relax.

Glutes can also improve aesthetics, health, strength, performance and play a crucial role in injury prevention.

You can use the exercises in this book to obtain a robust posterior, whether you're aiming to build muscular mass in your glutes for a shapely posterior or you want better functional strength for sports and intricate lifts.

The gluteus maximus provides most of the shape, power, and explosive posterior of the glutes, and it is majorly responsible for the movement of the thighs and hips.

However, all three gluteal muscles play important roles in the movement. The gluteus medius aids in hip rotation and stabilization, and the gluteus minimus helps to extend our hips.

Glute Isolation Exercises Vs. full body Exercises

We all know how important glutes are to the body, but why would you want to focus on them specifically? If you find yourself in an inactive lifestyle or a period of inactivity has left you with weakened hip extensors or glutes, or you just want to increase the size of your glutes and not your thighs, you should incorporate some of these glute isolation exercises into your workout routine.

Other workouts for the arms, shoulders, upper back, and lower body muscle groups such as the quads and hamstrings are also beneficial for overall health and fitness. Compound exercises that activate many muscles are often more challenging and a smarter and more precise method to work out quickly and make the most of your gym time, but isolation exercises are ideal if you want to focus on your glutes, especially if you don't need to expand the size of your tights as well.

In a leg press, for example, your foot position has an impact on which muscles are targeted during the exercise. Your glutes and hamstrings will be more targeted if your left and right feet are high up on the platform, but a lower foot position will ease the pressure off the hamstrings and glutes and put more strain on the quads.

7 Exercises to Target Your Glutes

Strong glutes are essential for a round booty, functional strength, and injury prevention at some of your body's most vulnerable joints. The glutes support your upper body and stabilize your knees and hips. Exercises for the glutes are especially crucial if you spend a lot of time sitting, as a sedentary lifestyle can cause them to atrophy.

You could spend a lot of time at the gym trying to work on your whole posterior, but if you want to focus on your glutes without having to build a mass of deadlift weight, the glute isolation exercises are the best way to do it.

Before you begin your glutes workout, you should ensure to focus on these glute isolation exercises we have listed in this book to make sure your calves and thighs aren't taking too much and robbing your glute muscle of the strength gain they would need.

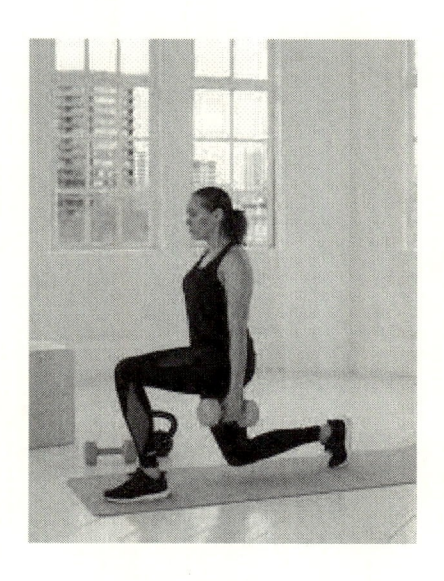

Stylist.co.uk

If you've ever done a leg work out, then you most likely know already familiar with a lunge. Lunges have long been known as one of the best exercises to increase the size of the gluteus maximus muscle.

A lunge is a pretty simple movement. It's critical to master the form of a traditional lunge because numerous lunge modifications are beneficial to glute, quad, and hamstring development.

Lunges are a bodyweight exercise that can be supplemented with dumbbells or resistance bands to give your glutes an extra workout. Start with your feet about hip-width apart in a standing position.

With your right foot, take a step forward. Make sure it's a little longer than your regular stride length. To accommodate the movement, lower your torso and continue lowering until your right thigh is parallel to the ground. Your left knee should be approximately parallel to the ground. By pressing through your right heel, return to the starting position.

The reverse deficit lunge is a great way to isolate and stimulate your glutes. You must stand on an elevated platform and stride backward with one leg in this movie. To accomplish one rep, lower into the same squat position as a traditional squat and then rise back to the starting position.

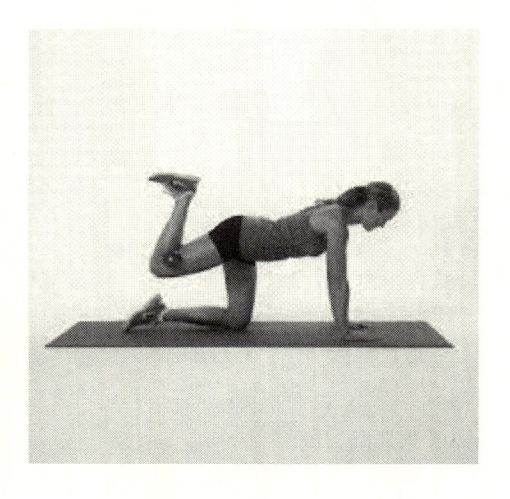

Popsugar.com

Donkey Kicks

Donkey kicks are one exercise that everyone can try at home, at the office, and just about anywhere you desire to do so. They are also one of the most common bodyweight exercises in which you could pair with a resistance band. Although the starting position may be a bit awkward, the donkey kickback is similar to the standard push-up. To start, support your upper body with your palms, ensure that they are flat on the ground directly under your shoulder, but unlike the conventional push-up, your lower body would be supported by your knees. Your knees should be bent at approximately a 90-degree angle.

For people who have problems with their knees but still want to add the donkey kick to their workout routine, they should place a yoga mat or some other kind of surface with a pad to protect the knees. They can the donkey kick as part of their wrap-up or stretch routine, they could, but you can also throw it in the main part of a bodyweight routine too.

Squeeze your glutes and send any of your legs backward as you straighten out the knee. At the top of this motion, by doing, you should have a line from the heel of the leg in motion to the top of your head. Return to the starting position and keep going through all your reps on one side before switching to the other leg.

Donkey kicks might seem so basic, but they are a great way of building strength in the gluteus maximus and for more stability in general.

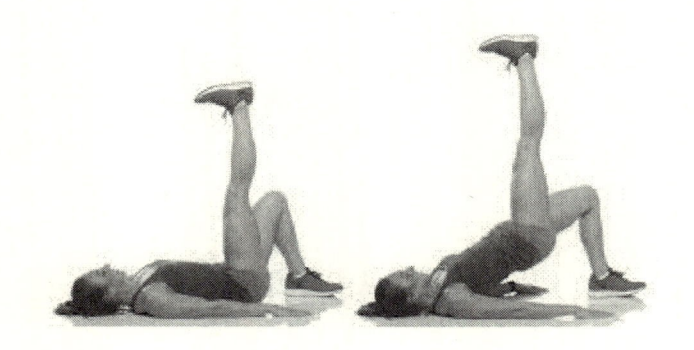

julielohre.com

Single-Leg Glute Bridge

For the glute bridge variation, you would focus on your gluteus maximus and medius. The trick is to add a single leg movement; you would also have the opportunity to give each leg more work out. Of course, this might ruin your workout plan and would cost you more time during your routine, but this bodyweight exercise isn't complicated that you always add it to a home routine also, in order to avoid wasting valuable gym time. During this technique, your hip adductors, quadriceps, hamstrings, and core muscles will all be activated, but because the major focus is on the two larger gluteal muscles, try wrapping a resistance band around your legs above the knee to make it even more difficult. To begin, lay on your back and bend your knees so that your feet' soles are flat on the ground. Ensure you keep both your hands at your sides, palms down. Raise your right or left leg into the air, keeping the knee straight. After that, clench your glutes together and lift your hips till a straight line runs from your neck to your lower knee. Hold that position for a few seconds before returning to the starting position. Then, carefully move your weight on the other leg after each single-leg exercise to receive an even workout on all sides of your body.

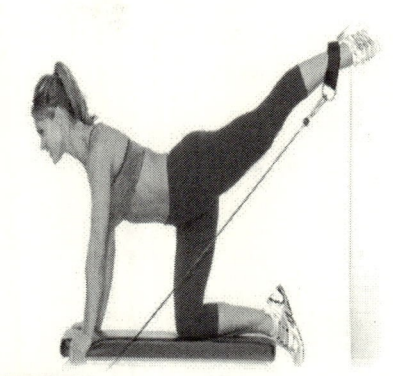

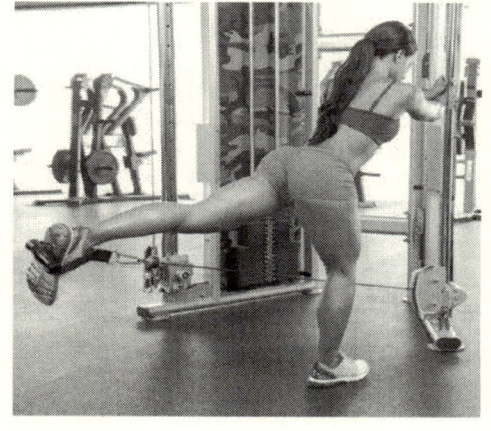

Skimble.com
ammfitness.co.uk

Glute Kickbacks

The gluten kickback is another single-leg exercise; it can be performed with either a pulley machine or a band with strong resistance, which can be secured to an anchor point. The resistance band is to help those who are working from home or at work. A heavy desk or table is ideal for holding one end of the band. The kickback ensures that all three glute muscles are activated. However, if you are using a pulley machine, place the pin where you desire in the weight plate and secure the Velcro strap around your right ankle. To garner stability, ensure you lean forward and place your right hand on a vertical bar or object. Ensure to hinge at the hips rather than rounding your back when leaning forward. Although your body won't make a 90-degree angle, your torso should be nearly parallel to the ground. Maintain a hip-width distance between your feet. Raise your right leg behind you now that you're in the starting position. Continue to do so until your right leg is parallel to your body. Some people can go a little higher, but the goal here is to maintain a straight line.

Hold the right leg in the highest position for 1–2 seconds before returning it to the beginning position. Make sure each side of your body gets the same number of reps.

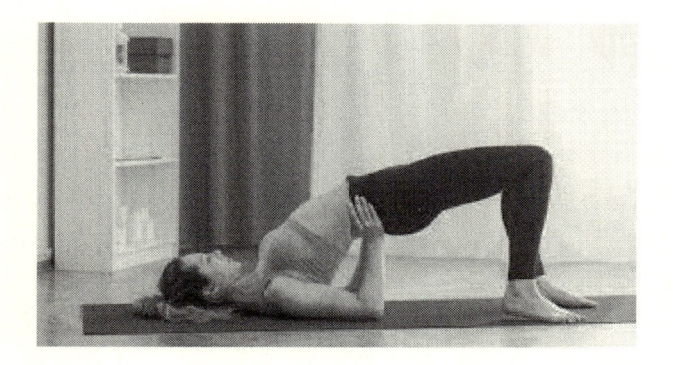

Healthline.com

Hip Thrust

The hip thrust is extremely similar to the glute kickback discussed earlier. Both exercises focus on hips elevation. The glute kickback and the hip thrust require elevation of the hips using glute strength, but the hip thrust is done with an elevated surface, while a glute kickback is done with the shoulders resting on the floor. The additional elevation of the hip thrust gives your glutes room to move through a larger range of motion. This exercise can be done on a sturdy bench, chair, or table as long as it isn't too high off the ground. You should be able to rest the back of your head on the elevated surface and lift your buttocks off the ground with your feet flat on the ground. You'll be robbing yourself of a large component of this workout if the bench or chair is too high since your glutes won't be able to sink as much. Try sitting in front of an elevated surface of your choice. As you sit, rest the back of your head on the surface. Place your feet on the ground shoulder width part from themselves, then slightly lift your butt off the ground to get to the starting position. To execute the exercise, begin by engaging your core and move glutes to ensure that your hips are lifted, and your torso is flat. Hold and squeeze your glutes at the top during motion and then return to the starting position. For additional difficulty, place and hold a barbell over your lap.

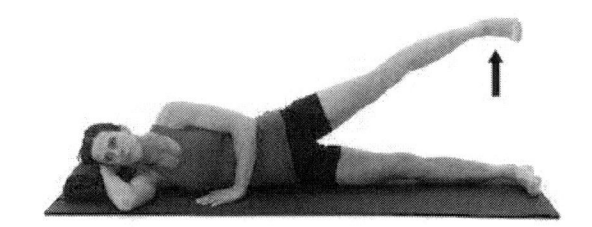

Basd.net

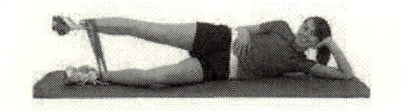

Performancehealthacademy.com

Side-Lying Hip Abductions

While they might not be as effective as full-body exercises like the Romanian deadlift, hip abductions are nonetheless great moves for targeting the glutes specifically. They're easy to do and offer plenty of activation for the gluteus medius and minimus.

Lie on your side with both legs spread out for a typical hip abduction workout. One leg should be on top of the other in this position. You can keep your hands tucked in or use your elbow to support your upper body as needed. Raise the top leg as high as possible and then lower it. Before rotating to the other side, finish all of your reps on that side. Although this is commonly thought of as a warm-up or novice move, many continue to make mistakes by going too fast or allowing their bodies to become out of alignment.

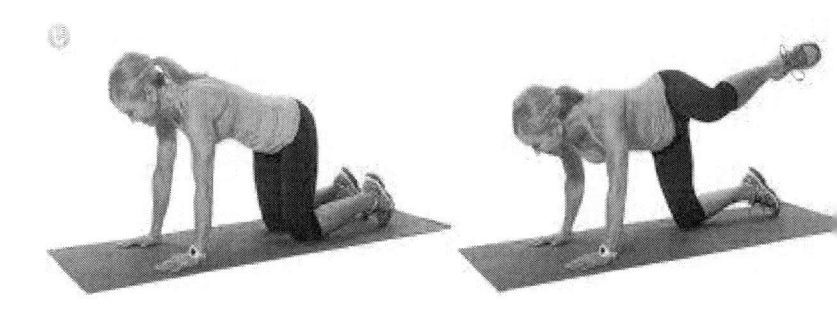

Gethealthyu.com

Fire Hydrant

Asides from its odd name, the fire hydrant is similar to donkey kicks, but it would need a lot more lateral movement, which is great for improving the gluteus medius. This exercise also improves your ability to move your side-by-side motion during exercise.

Starting position is identical to that of donkey kicks. Make sure your hands are just beneath your shoulders, and your knees are at a 90-degree angle when you get down on your hands and knees. In this fire hydrant move, the angle is more important than it was in the donkey kicks.

Raise your right leg out to the side without losing the 90-degree angle in your right knee once you're in the beginning position. If you experience any pain, don't try to raise your right leg higher at first. You're not trying to get your leg parallel to your chest like in previous exercises; instead, just get it as high as you can comfortably.

Ensure you lower the right legs and complete all your reps on each side before moving to the next. This exercise alongside the donkey glutes would help provide lateral strength and build your glutes.

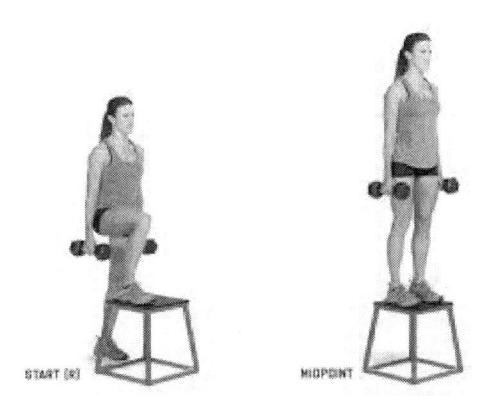

Velopress.com

The Step Up

The step-up is a unilateral leg exercise that works the gluteus maximus (hip extension), gluteus medius and minimus (hip and knee stabilization), and quadriceps. This exercise is beneficial for developing unilateral strength, correcting any imbalances, and increasing glute strength and hypertrophy. It's worth noting that the higher the step up, the more the hip flexion there is - this might lead to more demand on your glutes extending to the hips.

To begin, grab a pair of dumbbells and hold them at your sides. You can also hang them from the front rack or from the ceiling. Place one foot firmly in the box's middle, ensuring that your hip crease is below the knee. You can adjust the depth of the step up to target the glutes and/or quadriceps more effectively. Stand up with the front leg without springing off the grounded leg, keeping control at the top of the box while fully extending the hip and knee. To make it more challenging, don't put your ground foot on top of the box. This will put your unilateral stability, balance, and strength to the test.

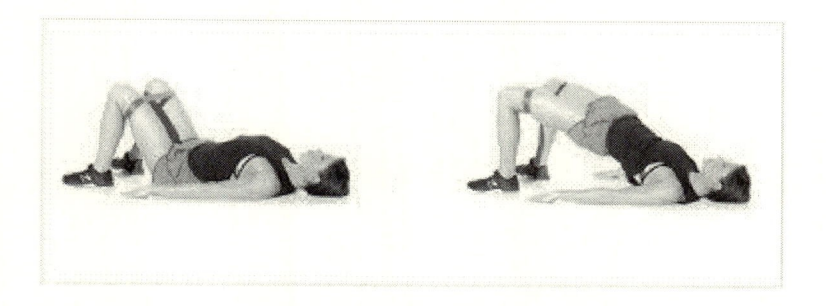

ammfitness.co.uk

Banded Glute Bridge

The banded glute bridge reinforces strength on the glutes. To get into the starting position, lay down with your knees bent, feet flat on the floor, and arms by sides on the floor with a resistance band around your thighs. Engage your core, then press into your heels and clench your glutes to elevate your hips to the ceiling while maintaining tension on the band. Before descending to begin, hold the position for a second. That's one rep; repeat for a total of 15 reps before moving on to the next exercise. (You should accomplish at least three reps.) Rest for up to one minute once you've completed all of your movements. Then do it three more times for a total of four rounds.

Why Your Glutes Aren't Growing Even After Training

The very first thing you should know before you begin your workout is to activate your glute. If not, you won't see the result, no matter how hard and long you work out. A simple stand-up or walk up the staircase utilizes your quads, but your glutes, on the other hand, you don't use as much every day, and the inactivity causes them to fall asleep, and you need to learn how to use them again.

Asides from the need to warm up their glutes, most women, in a bid to increase their glutes, focus so much energy on their legs and thighs instead of their butt and glute region. Focusing on a routine that focuses on both the thighs and butt would make you work twice as hard, and in most cases, you won't get your desired result. As earlier discussed, isolating your glutes would give your desired result.

What You Should Consider Before You Start Your Routine

It's possible that even after your training, your glutes might still not grow the way you want them to. You should put into these strategies listed below so as to understand what you should consider important and focus on in order to build around voluptuous and strong posterior.

- Training Capacity

We need to HYPERTROPHY (raise the size of) our glutes in order to develop them. This is simple to achieve if we train frequently and at a moderate weight. If you worked your glutes HARD once a week and had to recuperate for a whole week, this isn't going to help you build your glutes at all. Although it's a fantastic thing to train, if you train too frequently, you won't receive enough rest for your muscles to expand, making it difficult for them to grow. Simultaneously, if you exercise seldom and miss every opportunity to strike, you could do it for more than a year without changing anything. If you get a mix of these rarely exercising and exercising too hard: you require longer recovery, or not, and by the time you hit that muscle group again, you've lost the opportunity to cause more muscle damage for hypertrophy's sake.

Bear in mind that hypertrophy is got the size of your glutes increased in size, and the only way you could do so is by training those muscles over and over again with ample time for recovery. So, one hard session every week won't cut it out, neither would it grow those glutes. A minimum of time of 2 to 4 times a week would help give the required strength your glute needs to grow.

- **Exercise Selection**

There are a vast number of exercises that can do wonders for the growth of your glutes; however, not every form of exercise that works for the next person would work for you. The aim of this exercise is to grow your glutes and not a show of power between your gym buddies. So, why not attend a proper consultation and find the right exercise for your body type. The aim is to be able to squeeze and feel your glutes during the majority of your reps. And most exercises will have a dominant muscle group. However, there'll be some interplay with other muscle groups at some stage. Be sure to take note of what works for you.

- **Progressive Overload**

Progressive Overload is when a muscle area is subjected to a larger stimulus (tempo, load, reps and sets, rest periods) than it was previously. As your muscles become stronger and more acclimated to movement patterns, you will need to adjust these to achieve greater results. Paying attention to your biofeedback and workouts is the quickest approach to know when you should apply progressive Overload. You may want to find a middle ground, change your workout or simply do the same workout with intermittent breaks, at a slower tempo, half ranges, or simply less rest or do more sets and reps when the weight you began with now feels very easy to do.

- **Food consumption**

Your diet is also very important; neglecting your diet while training is threading on a dangerous path. Asides from that, you can also grow your glutes by focusing on the quality of food you take rather than on the right number of calories. Inculcating the right diet and focusing on the right quality of food would definitely set you on the right path.

Some common mistakes people make about their food consumption are.

- Not eating enough protein.
- Eating a lot of sweet and trigger foods.
- Eating too much soy and gluten.
- Inadequate sleep.
- Unregulated eating (under-eating and overeating)

Warm-up your Glutes Before Training

Don't start your glute workout without first doing some mobility work for the love of all things injury prevention. Sure, several of the best glute workouts above are performed solely with bands but don't make the mistake of utilizing heavy bands as warm-ups. When done correctly (slow, steady, deliberate, and possibly with a higher-resistance band), there's nothing like it.

CHAPTER FOUR

THE SRA CURVE FOR GLUTE TRAINING

This chapter will enlighten you on what the S.R.A. curve is about and how the S.R.A. curve is an integral factor when training your glutes. Let's get right into it.

What is S.R.A.?

The Stimulus Recovery Adaptation (S.R.A.) is a complex system. The stimulus is the exercise, as well as how long you exercise for. After the stimulus (workout session), a breakdown happens. The level of this breakdown is often dependent on how difficult the exercise is and your capacity to adapt to this exercise. For instance, the level of breakdown that happens when a beginner works out would be longer than when an expert does the same exercise.

The recovery process (the R in S.R.A.) is based on how large the duration of the breakdown is. If the breakdown process is huge, then there is a chance that the recovery process will be restricted. The last part is the Adaptation (the A in S.R.A.). Adaptation is often determined by the recovery process and is based on if the body has what it takes for Adaptation. It is at this stage that protein and nutrients come to play. With the right amount of protein, the body becomes well-fortified for Adaptation.

The S.R.A. has different subsystems. These subsystems include the muscle, the nervous system, and the Tendons/ligaments. However, for this chapter's purpose, I'm only going to be focused on the muscle S.R.A.

Muscle S.R.A.

Muscle S.R.A. is the major concept that determines the frequency of your glutes training. It focuses on how frequently you should train your glutes to achieve the best results when growing your booty.

The Muscle S.R.A. Curve

The S in the muscle S.R.A. represents the stimulus. And it's where your muscle breakdown to grow. After this breakdown, your body grows the muscle that has been broken down, and it is at this stage, the recovery stage occurs. After your body has built back this muscle, it becomes well strengthened to prevent subsequent breakdown, which happens when the muscle becomes larger than it originally was. This stage is often called the adaptation process. With the adaptation process, your body is trained to have a stronger resistance to future breakdown (stimulus).

However, because the body has become more resistant to stimulus, it requires a stronger force to break down. However, if the force is too strong, it could affect the recovery and the adaptation process. This is doing too much or too strong exercises all at once. When you do this, it could have a negative impact on the growth of your glutes; rather than help you grow your glutes, it hampers its growth.

Muscle Protein Synthesis

Muscle protein synthesis is where the recovery and adaptation process happen. During the S.R.A. curve, the muscle protein synthesis stage is heightened. When muscle protein synthesis goes back to the baseline, the recovery and adaptation process is finalized. This has proven to be the best time to brace your muscle again to begin the S.R.A. curve again.

How long should you train your muscles?

The short answer to how long you should train your muscles is when the muscle S.R.A. is completed. If you train your muscles too often, your muscle may diminish in size over time because you will constantly exercise before the muscle S.R.A. gets completed. If you train less often than required, there is a high chance that you will not reach the crest of the muscle S.R.A. curve. The best is to train your muscles after the recovery and adaptation stage to get the right results.

How long does it take for the Glute S.R.A. to get finalized?

Based on research, your muscle protein synthesis can be heightened for about 72 to 96 hours, which is about 3 to 4 days. The glutes muscle group takes at most 72 to 96 hours which is between 3 to 4 days, to finalize the muscle S.R.A. curve. So how long exactly should you wait between glute workout sessions? Well, the waiting period is dependent on the type of glute exercise and the process of your glute exercise.

Let's discuss the glute exercise below:

Muscle S.R.A. Exercise

Generally, when trying to grow your glutes. Exercises like hip thrusts, lunges, deadlifts, step-ups, and so on come into play. However, some exercises take longer to complete the muscle S.R.A. than others. So, the duration differs. There are basically four types of exercises that determine how long the muscle S.R.A. would take. Check them out below:

1. **Muscle Activity**

Muscle activity is similar to muscle tension, which is basically how your muscles get stimulated to grow. Your muscle's growth is based on your recovery and adaptation stage. If your muscle is highly activated, then your muscle tension is going to be high. However, if the muscle activation is low, then your muscle tension is going below. The recovery time for low muscle tension is usually short, while the recovery time for high muscle tension is often low.

2. **Range of Motion**

The Range of Motion is also called R.O.M. When your workout makes your muscle through a large R.O.M., your muscle will work more. The higher the training volume, the longer the duration of your recovery process. This means the exercises that take a larger Range of Motion usually require a longer recovery and adaptation process.

3. Emphasis on eccentrics

Heavy eccentric breakdowns have proven to break down your muscles than concentric activities. People who undergo heavy concentric movements usually take shorter days to recover, while people who undergo heavy eccentric movements take longer days to recover. One of the popular glute exercises that features an emphasis on eccentrics is the full squat. The full squats contain being in charge while your movement goes down and heightening the tension on the glutes in the process. Exercises like Band Hip thrusts only cause high tension at the top; then, as the movement goes lower, the tension on the glutes reduces.

4. Muscle Length at Peak Tension

Exercises that require hard work on the muscles when they are lengthened often result in increased breakdown of the muscles compared to when they are shortened. If you fire the muscles greatly when they are lengthened, there will be an increased breakdown, and the recovery process will take longer. However, if you increase the tension when they are shortened, then the recovery process will take a shorter S.R.A. curve.

Applying the four aspects to the glute's exercises:

Exercises like full squats usually take a longer duration to recover from because they require average glute activity. It transports the glutes to a large Range of Motion and places prominence on the eccentric phase, which is located at the eccentric phase 3. At this phase, there is peak tension whenever the glutes are lengthened. Due to this, there is an increased muscle breakdown, and because there is an increased muscle breakdown, the recovery process takes more time and, subsequently, a long adaptation phase. And as expected, the S.R.A. takes a longer period to get finalized because of the long recovery and adaptation phase, usually about 3 to 4 days.

The barbell hip thrust, for example, is an activator type of exercise. This exercise requires a short recovery phase because its Range of Motion (R.O.M.) is small-scale. Because the tension is at its highest when the glutes are lessened. The Barbell hip thrust comes with a massive eccentric phase. And because the tension on the muscle is at its highest during the adaptation phase, the muscle builds bigger during the adaptation phase on the S.R.A. curve. Due to this, the S.R.A. curve takes a fairly long duration cycle to get completed. And this could take about 2 to 3 days.

The Band Side Walks is a pumper exercise type, and it comes with a little Range of Motion (R.O.M.), so the movement on the glutes is short. Due to this, there is tension at its highest when the muscle is reduced. Therefore, the

S.R.A. curve duration takes about 1 to 2 days to get finalized.

Muscle Hypertrophy

Muscle hypertrophy is the increase and development of your muscle cells. It is the increase in your muscular size that basically happens when you exercise. And lifting weight has been the most common way to achieve growth in any part of your muscle, including your glutes.

There are 3 major ways to achieve muscle hypertrophy. Let's discuss them below:

1. Mechanical Tension

Mechanical tension is the type of tension that is generated when you use a heavy load and undergo an exercise between a range of motion at a particular time. The duration of time the muscle spends tensioned is enabled by the heavy load you use (this could be a dumbbell, barbell, and so on) generates a mechanical tension on your muscle. The more time you spend exercising using a heavy load, the higher the mechanical tension. However, when trying to grow your muscle, tension isn't all that is needed. To reach the state of hypertrophy, your muscle needs to undergo a full Range of Motion (R.O.M.).

2. Muscle Damage

Muscle damage is an integral part of the hypertrophy process. And it usually happens during resistance and strength training exercises. Eccentric and concentric exercises are known to cause muscle damage. A significant type of muscle damage is the D.O.M.s (Delayed Onset of Muscle Soreness) is a popular type of muscle damage that happens during workout sessions. The delayed onset of Muscle Soreness comes as a result of mini tears around the muscle. Although both the eccentric and concentric contractions can result in muscle damage, eccentric contractions have proven to cause increased damage of the muscle than concentric contractions. This is why muscle builders often introduce negative reps in their workout routine. Negative reps happen when you lift extra weight than you normally would. This could range from 30-40% more weight.

For example, let's say you want to do negative reps on the bench press. So, if you do a bench press of 150kg when you are by yourself, then you can add an extra 30kg on the bar for your negative rep, which makes it about 180kg.

After this, you put yourself in the bench press position, and your partner helps you unpack the bar, and you lower the weight on your chest slowly for about 2 to 3 seconds. Once the weight gets to the lowest point, your partner helps you carry the weight up, removing the extra 30kg bar you included initially. After this, you press the bar back to the top, and you do this repeatedly.

The reason bodybuilders do negative reps is that it enables them to lift heavier weight. The heavier the weight you lift, the more muscle damage, which helps you get stronger at a faster period of time which helps your glute muscle grow bigger. Negative reps enable you to put extra pressure on your muscle than regular training, which helps to grow stronger glute muscles.

3. Metabolic Stress

Metabolic stress is one of the most important factors that enable hypertrophy. To grow your glute muscles, you would have to put your muscles under stress to adjust. The stress corresponds to the weight of the load you place on your muscle, and the heavier the load is, and the longer the exercise duration is, the higher the stress that leads to an increase in muscle growth.

Lifting weight for increased repetitions helps you build your glute muscles. When you perform resistance training, you experience the burn and the pump when you reach increased reps, which is often accompanies by a short rest time. During each rep, several actions take place. Your muscle continuously contracts and relaxes, and blood pooling takes place around your muscle. As a result of this, the blood that flows to the muscle is restricted, and there is barely enough blood to fuel the muscle during the consistent contractions that take place.

There is a massive development of metabolites such as hydrogen ions and lactate as a result of this. And the stress on the muscle is followed by an anabolic effect that results in an increased hormonal reaction from your body.

Hypertrophy occurs as a result of these three major factors: Mechanical tension, Muscular damage, and metabolic stress. When these three factors are put together, there is an anabolic effect that is generated by molecular signaling. The anabolic effect that occurs helps trigger muscle growth. It also helps to maximize protein synthesis that is responsible for muscle repair.

Glute Muscle Exercises

Now that you understand what the hypertrophy stage is as well as the mechanisms responsible for this stage, what kind of exercises should you do consistently to undergo the three mechanisms discussed above to grow your glute muscles? There three major exercises: the stretchers, the activators, and the pumpers. I will discuss the 3 exercise types below:

1. Stretcher exercises

Stretcher exercises help bring your glute muscles to a large Range of Motion (R.O.M.). It places emphasis on the eccentric phase, and the peak tension occurs when the glutes muscles are lengthened. As a result of this, a muscle breakdown occurs. Stretcher exercises have a longer recovery period and take about 4-6 days to get back to the baseline, depending on your level of training. Stretching your glutes helps relieve the tightness in your muscle and enhance your range of motion. Stretcher exercises help relieve the discomfort that comes with back pain, pain in your buttocks, pelvic area, and knee area. It also helps increase your flexibility and mobility and enhance your Range of Motion.

Why should you perform stretcher exercises for your glutes?

Glute exercises are great if you are trying to warm up before your workout session. This helps increase your blood flow into your glute muscles and prep them up for the upcoming workout session.

Stretching your glutes with stretcher exercises is also important after every workout session. It enhances flexibility and mobility and promotes a better exercise performance for your next workout session. Stretcher exercises are also great to help stretch your glutes when you notice you've sat for too long. Stretching your glutes exercises consistently can help reduce the stiffness in your muscle area. Certain stretcher exercises like sumo deadlift, Romanian deadlift, lunge, and side-lying hip abduction help strengthen your glutes muscles, enhance your balance and improve your body composition.

When should you perform stretcher exercises for your glutes?

You should perform stretcher exercises for your glutes at the beginning of your workout session to prep your body for the exercises you want to perform. Dynamic stretching exercises that involve performing stretching exercises at a spot or at a slow pace can help increase blood flow into your workout. An example is performing squats but at a slow pace, which involves slowing moving your buttocks up and down to warm up your glute muscles. You can also perform stretcher exercises at the end of your workout sessions to increase your flexibility and improve your performance for subsequent pieces of training.

Stretcher Exercise Types for Your Glutes

There are different stretcher exercises you can perform for your glute muscles. The most popular stretcher exercises include sumo deadlift, Romanian deadlift, lunge, and side-lying hip abduction. Let's discuss them below:

1. Sumo Deadlift

The sumo deadlift is one of the most incredibly effective stretcher exercises that increases your glutes muscles flexibility and strengthens your muscles. The sumo deadlift is done with different types of equipment. But the most popular equipment that works best with sumo deadlift is a barbell. Here is a step-by-step guide on how to perform the sumo deadlift.

Step 1

Begin your sumo deadlift by making your feet wider than your shoulder width. Point your toes forward and make your legs wide enough to enable you to place your arms in between your knees. Ensure to keep your thighs and knees correspond with your toes.

Step 2

Bend your body and hold the barbell. Then, begin to generate tension by dragging the bar and shoving the feet on the ground. Brace your core and straighten your back and ensure to place your shoulders directly above the bar.

Step 3

Drag the bar up as you push through your legs. And ensure to place your bar close to your body to end your movement.

Step 4

Place the bar to the ground after you've completed the movement. You can perform this exercise as repetitively as you desire.

Activator Exercises

Activator exercises have a smaller range of movement along with a peak tension when the glutes muscles have been greatly shortened. Activator exercises can be maximized with a heavy-loaded eccentric phase. This means when you control the weight when you go down, there is mechanical tension and, subsequently, muscle damage. The recovery process of activator exercises takes about 2 to 3 days to return to the baseline.

Glute activation exercises help stimulate your glute muscles. Activator exercises help to contract your glutes. When you perform glute exercises, you should feel a "burn" in your glute. However, it's important you don't overdo activation exercises, so they do not leave you exhausted, especially if you plan to perform a lower body workout session after a glute activator exercise.

Why should you perform activator exercises?

Glute activator exercises help you activate your glute muscles so your glutes muscles can perform better during your workout sessions. Activator exercises help improve the strength of your glute muscles through effective movement that boosts your muscle performance. Glute muscle exercises enable you to target your glute muscles effectively to give you enhanced performance when strengthening and growing your glute muscles.

How frequently should you perform activator exercises?

Performing glute exercises every day helps keep your glutes muscles active, especially if your lifestyle involves sitting down for long. By keeping your glutes active, you are less prone to the strains and tears that come with inactive glutes.

The Best Activator Exercises for Your Glutes

To effectively activate your glutes, you need to perform glute isolation exercises. Exercises such as squats might not be effective at targeting your glute muscles because they are compound movements. So, they will most likely activate other areas of your body, such as your legs, and not target your glutes specifically. Below are the top exercises you can perform to grow your muscles the best way possible.

1. *Front Plank with Hip Extension*

Step 1

1. Put yourself in a plank position with your trunk, hips, and knees aligning
2. Raise your left leg from the ground, bend the knee of your left leg and stretch your hip by raising the heel in the direction of the ceiling. Maintain this position for a second and go back to the parallel position for about a second.
3. Then, repeat this on your second leg as many times as you want.

2. **Single leg squat**

How to do it:

- Begin by standing with your arms stretched to the front
- Balance one of your legs with your opposite leg. Then stretch out the straight leg in front for as much as you can.

- Squat as low as you can while keeping your leg raised.

- Straighten your back and keep your knees in the same direction as the supporting foot.

3. *Side Plank Abduction with Dominant Leg up*

How to do it:

- Lie on your side and place your body at the lowest part of your foot. Then, raise your hips in the air, create a straight line from your ankles to your shoulders.

- Ensure to keep your torso stable, then lift your leg and avoid bending your knees while you do so. Ensure to keep your hips in the air. Then go back to your starting position.

Pumper Exercises

Pumper exercises have a small range of motion and involve low activities on the glute. There is peak tension when the muscles are shortened. However, due to the consistent tension that occurs, pumper exercises are excellent for generating metabolic stress. Pumper exercises are called so because they make the muscle look pumped. Pumper exercises take between 1-2 days ballpark to recover at baseline. Pumper exercises include banded lateral walk, banded seated abduction, and elevated Glute Bridge. Etc.

Why should you perform pumper exercises for your glutes?

Pumper exercises are great for strengthening your glutes. They help with general body shaping, so you can achieve a good booty shape when you do the bumper exercises right. Pumper exercises also help burn your calories efficiently and also improve your muscle by toning your muscles.

Pumper Exercise Types

Below are the top pumper exercises that help improve your glutes muscles the best way.

1. Banded Lateral Walk

How to do it:

- Place a looped resistance band around your legs in your knee area. Then, stand with your feet together.

- Put your back in a flat position, and keep abs engaged, then shove your hips behind and lower your knees. After this, bend your body into a squatting position, then shift your weight in the direction of your heels.

- Maintain the squatting position and lift your hips a number of inches up. Step your right foot to the right side and bend your hips completely.

- Lift your hips a number of inches higher and place your left foot together with your right side. Then, bend your body completely and ensure to keep the tension in the band intact, so your knees don't go in.

- Do the same for the opposite sides and perform the same reps on both sides.

2. Banded seated abduction

How to do it:

- Get seated on the floor with your elbows relaxed on a chair and bench at your back. Then, put a booty band around the lowest part of your thighs. Seat tall to straighten your spine. Do not droop.
- Spread your knees to any of your sides and shove your booty band to maintain resistance.
- Go as far as possible, then place your knees together.
- Do this at least 20 times.

Addressing Split Body workout

While a full-body workout engages all of your muscle groups in one session, splits workouts are created to separate your muscle groups from one another. Splits help you make the most of your muscle growth and lessen your rest days. When you commit a day to one of your muscle groups, such as your glutes, you can target this muscle group efficiently from different angles, thereby maximizing the growth of that muscle. Splits involve rotating movements, such as the push, pull, and leg movements, after which you take a rest day after you've completed the three movements. For example, you can dedicate some days to your upper body muscles and other days to your lower body muscle then, take a rest day.

How to Turn Up Your Gains

Increasing how often you train helps increase your weekly training volume. Volume is the complete amount of work you do. So, if you increase the amount of weight you lift, you can increase your volume for more gains. Increasing the amount of time, you train helps increase your volume so you can gain more.

In this chapter, I discussed the Muscle S.R.A. curve, the top mechanisms involved in the muscle S.R.A. curve, as well as the different glutes muscle exercises you can do to grow your muscles the best way. In the next chapter, I will provide an effective glute program that gives the best outcome.

CHAPTER FIVE

A GLUTE PROGRAM THAT WILL PRODUCE THE BEST RESULTS

No one wants a magical transformation of their glutes. However, everyone would like to get the most of their glute's exercise. The first thing that must be done whenever you decide to grow your glutes is to find the right set of exercises that would stimulate the glutes. Exercise experts have determined the right amount of movement and activity that could produce the muscles through electromyography or EMG, so you could focus on the right way to activate the muscles.

How does the EMG work? When the glutes muscles contract, it lets off a signal. Those signals could be measured by electromyography. A machine hooked up to your body using simply stick pads on the skin. With these experts can fully comprehend the extent to which the muscles are working hard whenever you perform an exercise.

How Often Should You Train

The right amount of time dedicated to training and workout muscle growth is a controversial topic among fitness experts. Most experts think that training your muscles at least once a week is the best way to go about it (Hackett *et al.*, 2013).

Although a recent study concluded suggests that working your muscles twice a week had a higher result on hypertrophy compared to once per week (Schoenfeld et al., 2016).

However, modern lifters believe that training multiple times a week would put you at the edge for better results. Some contemporary lifters have also come forward to give perfect examples of when training multiple times works. To answer how often should one train their glute muscles, the short answer should be at least 2 to 6 times on an average weekly.

The long answer to this question would require that you read on to understand the various variables you would need to understand to fully optimize your ability, recovery process and the most effective frequency for your training. For appropriate training, you should realize that your intentions should be to focus on a specific matched volume frequency which might be more potent on your muscles than any other volume matched frequency because the distribution of the glute growth stimuli might become optimal throughout a week's training in one case and not in the other.

In simple terms, this means that spreading out 15 sets of muscle training over several workouts in a week can be more effective in growing your muscles than doing a complete 15 sets in one workout session. Some fitness expert believes that there is a maximum level of growth your muscles stimuli can experience in one workout session. For instance, if the maximum growth stimulus your muscles can experience would happen at seven sets, any other sets at this point would be considered as wasted efforts.

Logically, from the traditional bodybuilding split, which goes for muscle training for one time per week, most of these 15 sets would be wasted or counterproductive as the extra sets might hamper your recovery from the growth stimulus. And full-body routines typically spread the 15 sets out over several days. This may result in fewer wasted sets per workout.

Understanding the Glute Growth

The muscle SRA curve

The SRA muscle is the fundamental principle that serves as a guide as to how often you should train your glutes and methods by which you could grow them as fast as you desire. The S here stands for stimulus; during your workout session, your body breaks down the muscle, which is the stimulus for growth. As a result of this, the muscles functional size begins to decrease. The functional size is the only part that is still able to contract. Because the body has broken down the muscles, it would begin to start rebuilding the broken-down muscles; this process of rebuilding is called RECOVERY, the R in SRA. After the body has gone through all of these processes, it begins to build up resistance that would prevent further breakdown of the muscle. The resistance is done by building the muscle into a bigger size than it was originally. This process is called ADAPTATION, the A in SRA. The muscle has built a stronger level of resistance to a future stimulus.

This is known as Adaptation, the A in SRA.

The muscle has grown more resistant to a future Stimulus (basically, a thicker wall needs a bigger straining to break it down).

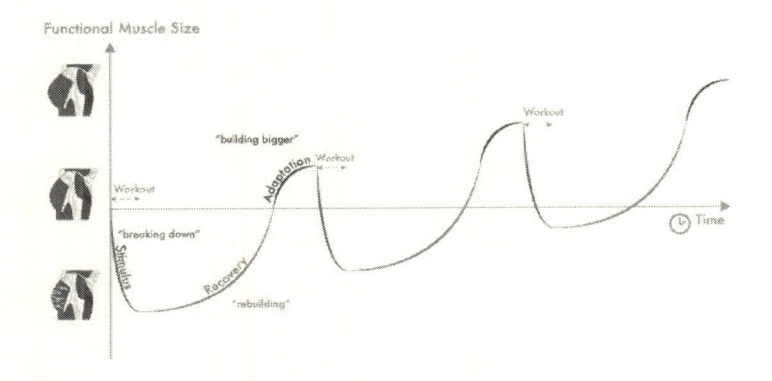

[source]

If the new workout routine or training is too hard, it might cause more harm than good. It could stall the process of recovery or adaptation.

Finally, the SRA principle doesn't apply to just your muscle. Other parts of the body also have the SRA curves, for instance, the muscles, which goes directly into the nervous system and connective tissues (such as muscle tendons).

When should you train again?

The answer to this question is answered from the Muscle SRA curve. As soon as the curve is completed, then you can begin your training again; however, you should note that each person's recovery and adaptation time is unique to them partly answers this question: when the muscle SRA curve is completed.

It is important you understand when your SRA muscle cycle is complete so as not to Train too frequently because the muscle will actually *decrease* in functional size over time. As a result of you constantly stimulate the muscles before your adaptation and recovery have been completed. Training too infrequently would make you unable to fully utilize the peak period of the SRA curve as a starting point to further your muscle growth.

Type of Glute Exercises

Stretchers

Stretchers are a form of high-intensity glute exercises. They are usually performed between 3-4 days' rest activators. Examples include lunges, weighted squats, and deadlifts.

Activators

Activators are moderate-intensity glute exercises, and you'll need between the 2-3 days' rest between stretchers. Examples include weighted hip thrusts, cable kickbacks and glute bridges, and cable pull through.

Pumpers

Pumpers are low-intensity glute exercises that you would need a day rest between pumpers. Examples are resistance band glute bridges, bodyweight squats, and resistance band crab walks.

Optimal Glute Training
Pumpers, Activators, and Stretchers
@strengthwithsam

Stretchers

Activators

Pumpers

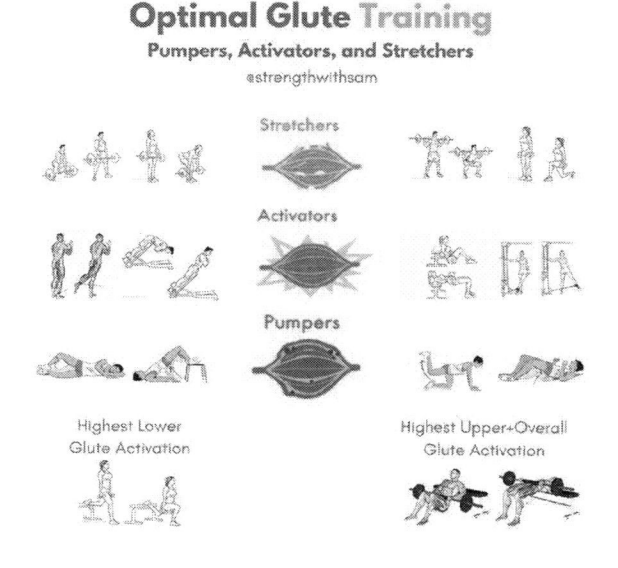

Highest Lower Glute Activation

Highest Upper+Overall Glute Activation

Pinterest.com

Muscle Protein Synthesis

Your protein synthesis is very important when it comes to the rebuilding and recovery of your muscle. Your muscles adaptation and recovery can only happen through muscle protein synthesis. During the course of the growth of the muscle and SRA curve, muscle protein synthesis is often increased.

And when the protein synthesis gets back to the baseline, the process of adaptation and recovery becomes complete. At this point, it is the perfect time to stimulate the muscles again if you want to kick start the muscle SRA curve.

How long does it take the Glute SRA curve to get completed?

As a result of the presence of the EMG to measure long term muscle protein synthesis structure, studies have shown that the muscles protein synthesis can stay high for a maximum period of 3 to 4 days (72 to 96 hours) as we know by now that the muscle protein synthesis is responsible for the fundamental rebuilding (recovery) and adaptation (growth) of muscles.

Now, to the muscle group of our interest: The Glutes.

It takes a maximum of 3 to 4 days for a muscular SRA curve to get completed. That means you shouldn't wait for 120 to 144 hours (5 to 6 days) between Glute workouts if you want them to grow as quickly as possible. How long should one wait before, here it would depend on some factors.

- The type of glute exercise and
- The glute training experience

Particularly for the glutes, there are a number of exercises used to stimulate, like the external rotations, hip abductions, squats, lunges, step-ups, and all of its variations, to name a few, they can all be used to stimulate the Glutes.

Some activities, however, may necessitate longer muscle SRA curves than others. Consider this scenario: On a regular day, you do four sets of Band Side Walks, and two days later, you do four sets of hard Bulgarian Split Squats. Is it true that the Glutes take the same amount of time to recover and adapt from these two training sessions? No because muscle repair and adaptation from hard Bulgarian Split Squats take a long time.

Why? Because there are four aspects of an exercise that influence the length of the muscle SRA curve.

Muscle Activity

Muscle tension is closely linked to muscle activation during a workout. When it comes to stimulating a muscle to grow, muscle tension is crucial. If you don't trust me, try practicing biceps curls to strengthen your Glutes (which show close to zero Glute activity).

A muscle grows by recuperating and adapting to a stimulus, as we all know. Low muscle tension low muscle activation, resulting in a minimal stimulus with a quick recovery time. Greater muscle tension results from high muscle activation, resulting in a larger stimulus with a longer recovery and adaptation period.

Range of motion

If an exercise allowed a muscle to go through a bigger range of motion than expected, the muscle would be required to do more work. Basically, muscular work is synonymous with muscle force, tension and distance. In most cases, the muscular work is usually referred to as training volume, which is an inappropriate name for it. In contrast, studies have shown that the heavier work (training volume) a muscle performs, the longer time it takes to recover. This indicates that exercises with a bigger Range of motion would take a longer time recovery and adaptation, probably because there would be more muscle breakdown due to the rise in heavy muscle work.

Emphasis on Eccentrics

Research has shown that heavy eccentrics helps in breaking down the muscles faster than heavy concentric movement. People who participate in these exercises took much longer to recover to their previous performance levels after the eccentrics. However, it took them only a day to recover from the concentric movement. A great example of glute exercises that focuses on the eccentrics would be the full squat. For the full squat, total control is gained while the weight is going down, while the pressure on the glutes increases gradually. Banded hip thrusts, on the other hand, are weightier on the top and would become increasingly lighter as you go lower.

This is because the resistance from the elastic band decreases. Without a doubt, it is understandable that the full squats place emphasis on the eccentric part of the movement, while the Band Hip Thrusts don't. As a result of this, the Squats would take longer to recover and adapt.

Muscle length at peak tension

Studies have also shown that applying pressure on your muscles when they are lengthened would cause more muscles breakdown than when they are shortened. As a result of these, it took a long time for the muscles to recover and adapt from the tension. For instance, if you participate in two different versions of the partial bicep curl, there would be peak tension in the biceps when it's lengthened. This would result in more muscle breakdown and a longer SRA curve. The other version would cause a peak tension when it's shortened, resulting in less muscle breakdown and a shorter SRA curve. For better understanding, let us apply these aspects to some glute exercise.

The Band Side Walks

The band sidewalk has a small range of motion, which gives a low average glute activity. When the muscle is shortened, then they show peak tension. Hence, the SRA curve would take a short while to complete (1-2 days). The band sidewalk would be categorized as a Pumper type of exercise. That is because the short range of motion and varying tension on the Glutes (band elastic resistance changes) allow for more reps to be performed, which causes a lot of "metabolic stress".

Barbell Hip Thrust

Because the range of movement for the barbell hip thrust is small, it would require a shorter time to recover from, and when the glutes are shortened, a peak tension occurs; however, the barbell hip thrust tremendously improves glutes activity with a heavily loaded eccentric phase (if you control the weight down, which a lot of people don't do). Higher muscles stimulate a bigger adaptation of the SRA curve. Because of this, the SRA curve takes a little longer time to complete (2-3 days). We could label the barbell hip thrust as an Activator type of exercise.

The full squat

Finally, the Full Squats, it would take longer to recover from; they allow moderate glute activity while placing emphasis on the eccentric phase, and the tension is created on the glutes when they are lengthened. With these, you would be left with a lot of muscle breakdown, which would require more time for recovery and adaptation. Hence resulting in a long time for the completion of the SRA curve (3-4 days). The full squat would be categorized as a stretcher type of exercise.

Exercises That Grow Your Glutes

Generally, larger muscles would take a longer time to recover, as the load of the volume and activity is done to inflict strain on the muscle, which makes the fatigue increase, although the glutes would not large muscles when compared to the muscles behind the leg and thighs, they are large enough to handle a large number of loads.

For this reason, it is important that you train the glutes in higher volumes and only a few times a week (eight to 15 total sets per session). In contrast, if you want to train, you train your glutes regularly (at least four times per week), you could dedicate time to doing four to eight sets per training session. This should be done without placing extra weight or stress on the glutes.

Below, we include the different times of glute exercise that could be done both at home and at work and two different glute workouts for acquiring mass.

Glute mass-building exercises (eccentric emphasis)

Below are some compound glute exercises that could foster high eccentric strength on the glutes one muscles, increasing the glute muscles hypertrophy and stress

Back squats

Back squats are known to be one of the most effective workouts for increasing the size of the quadriceps and glutes in the lower body. They're not an isolation exercise, but they can stimulate a lot of muscle mass and serve as an excellent basis for glute development.

Single-Leg Deadlift

The single led deadlift, just like the squat, activates the gluteus maximus and medius.

Start by standing tall with a dumbbell in your hand. Shift your weight to your left leg at the same time, bend your knees slightly. Forward with your upper body and reach for the ground with your arms. Thrust further to the ground with the dumbbells until your hands are hanging above your knees, then stand back up, ensure you do not touch your right leg to the ground throughout the period your left leg is active. Change sides and repeat the process with your right leg on the ground.

Front squats

Front squats, like back squats, can help you improve your legs and glutes. While the quadriceps are the primary muscle targeted, the back and glutes are also important throughout the activity.

Romanian deadlifts

Romanian deadlifts are a glute and hamstring-dominant exercise that can be utilized as a foundation for the development of the posterior chain (hamstrings, glutes, and back). This can also be done unilaterally for further muscle development and activation.

The Bulgarian split squat

For the Bulgarian split squat, the glutes are quite engaged, both in the eccentric phase for hip stability and control, as well as in deeper levels of hip flexion. Wider splits can also help you engage your hamstrings and glutes.

Lunges

Lunges of all kinds can help you grow your unilateral glutes, strengthen them, and improve hip/knee stability. Crossover lunges, reverse lunges, and walking lunges all impose a significant amount of stress on the glutes.

Glute Step-Up

This glute exercise contains a series of range movements. This motion means you get to work more on your fibre. You might, at some point, feel a little stretch at the bottom of the movement.

To get into the starting position, find a flat surface; the surface should be at least knee-high to step on. Place a foot on the top close to the edge, lean forward, and then push through that leg and lift your body up and step onto the surface with your other foot.

Stand upright at the top, then move back down with the same foot that you used in stepping up. At the end of each set, change the leg and perform the same number of reps on the other leg.

Glute Mass-Building Exercises (Concentric priority)

Below are some exercises which place a high priority on peak contractions at the end of the lifting phase, which can lead to an increase in glute activation and overall development

Hip Thrust

Hip thrusts are a great exercise for ensuring that there is a muscle contraction that is just enough for the high amount of metabolic stress that strengthens the muscles. Furthermore, this exercise is a form of glute isolation exercise and can be done with a high and low intensity, often to either load off or increase muscle damage.

The cable Pull-through

Just Like the hip thrust, the cable pulls through gives room for a lifter to maximally squeeze the glutes at the peak of each rep while also having increased time under tension as the cables constantly apply to load the glutes and hamstrings.

Quadruped Banded Hip Extension

The quadruped banded hip extension has proven to be an effective exercise at increasing the high amount of glutes activation and could be done easily with minimal loading using manual resistance, bands, or even exercise machines.

The Glutes Bridge

The Glute Bridge is a terrific technique to add increased range of motion and peak contraction exercises to your routine. It can be done unilaterally or bilaterally. This exercise can also help with any muscular imbalances or hip instability that may be preventing glute development and health.

Side-Lying Banded Leg Raise

Because they need less loading and can attack the glute on time under a tension basis, side-lying banded leg raises/lifts are a terrific method to finish a glute workout. They also improve hip function and mobility by increasing the glute's ability to shift the legs into abduction.

Band Sumo Walk

Although the lateral band walking exercise may appear (and feel) strange, it is an effective way to improve hip stability, strengthen your hips abductors (particularly the gluteus medius), and promote knee joint stability.

Side-Lying Hip Abduction

For the gluteus medius, which is the major muscle on the side of your hips. Side-lying hip abductions are major exercises to grow your glutes because they isolate the muscle. This move is often used to strengthen the gluteus medius. Start by lying on your side with your legs piled on each other. Place the hand on the top hip. Also, ensure your knees are placed straight, then lift your top leg straight up toward the ceiling, without bringing it forward or backward, then bring it back down to the other leg. Once you are done with that set, turn over and repeat with the other leg. You can make this exercise harder by putting a mini resistance band around your ankles.

With all of these in mind, you could apply this to your training schedule. Or you could make use of the schedule below for an increased glute size in thirty days.

- Monday: Lower Body Strength (Stretchers + Pumpers)
- Tuesday: Glutes (Activators + Pumpers)
- Wednesday: back + Chest + Glute Pump (Pumpers)

- Thursday: Legs + Glute Pump (Stretchers + Pumpers)
- Friday: Arms + glute Pump (Pumpers)
- Saturday: Glutes (Activators)

In this chapter, you have read about glute programs that you can try out for you to get the best results. If you follow your training plan diligently, you can get the best results you desire in 30 days. You can follow the recommended programs for each day in this chapter.

CHAPTER 6

EAT TO GROW YOUR BOOTY

Your diet and exercise are two of the most important factors for your overall health. Your body is a vehicle by which you carry out activities, and during your workout or training session, it serves as an engine that keeps you running. This means that how you treat and fuel your engine is super important. Eating the right food and taking proper fluid in the right quantity and at the right time is an important way by which you keep your engine charged up.

The consumption of sufficient food and fluids before and after exercise would help maintain a healthy balance of blood sugar and glucose during exercise and also help boost exercise performances and elevate recovery time.

It is important to find balance for your food and fluid intake during your workout session, and this can only be achieved when your body is well feed and hydrated during and after the exercise.

When it comes to putting your body through these rigorous faces that would build the muscles, you must always endeavor to fuel it with proper nutrition. By nutrition, this doesn't mean indulging in pre work out supplements. It is having a real, good and healthy meal or snacks. Basically, the kind of food you enjoy regularly and would most likely enjoy while you are trying to grow your glutes.

Consequently, your bodies' nutrition and exercise are two important factors that affect each other. This is because proper nutrition can provide strength to fuel your body during the exercises and at the same time help your body adapt, replenish and recover.

However, there is one common question on what to eat before and after exercising. This may be particularly relevant to people who exercise first thing in the morning. Now, understand that you do not have to adhere to a strict schedule, neither is there a hard and fast track to it, but you should have some relevant considerations in mind and do before and after your workout session. Even though it is worth it, figuring out what to eat before and after your workout can be such a struggle.

When it comes to a pre-workout meal, what you choose to put in your mouth is vital. This would determine how much strength your engine is running on. Of course, the food you eat after a workout is also important because refueling after a workout session would give your body the relevant nutrient to recover and replenish from the rigorous exertion and also help you build bigger and stronger muscles.

This means that being intentional about the food you eat before and after exercising would help prove the benefit of all your effort at building your glutes. What is the best pre work out snacks or meal? And what's best to eat after a workout? I recommend the meals and snacks below. Consider them a critical part of your training.

Before your exercise: charge up.

You must change yourself before any workout session; not fueling your engine up is like driving a car on an empty tank. You won't go far. You won't have enough energy to accelerate your training, and it would limit your ability to build your glute muscles.

Ideally, you must fuel up at least 2 hours before your workout starts by:

Hydrating yourself with water.

Consuming healthy carbohydrates such as whole-grain cereals (with low-fat or skim milk), whole-wheat toast, low-fat yoghurt, whole grain pasta, brown rice, fruits or vegetables.

Avoid saturated and heavy Protein because these types of meals would take time before digesting and, in the process, restrict your oxygen and the energy being delivered into your muscles.

However, if you have only a few minutes before you exercise, then you could take a piece of fruit, either an apple or a banana. The important thing here is to consume healthy and easily digestible carbohydrates, so do feel inactive or sluggish.

After: Refuel Your Tank.

After your workout, you should consider refueling with:

Fluids. Fluids, in this case, mean water. You must drink water to stay hydrated. However, you could sometimes choose 100% fruit juice. The ideal fruit juices are orange and apple, which provides bodily fluids.

Carbohydrates. During your workout, you burn many carbohydrates, which is the main means of energy for your muscles each time your exercise. Eating carbohydrates minutes after your workout can help your muscles store up energy to help in recovery.

Protein. Fortify your meals with proteins to help repair worn out tissues and grow your muscles.

The Effect of Junks on Your Muscle Growth

By now, you understand that every meal you consume allows your muscle to grow or derail your fitness goal. Fast food junks are the major tranquillizer to your muscle-building goal; they would put your efforts in vain.

Your diet or meal plan should contain low calorie and high protein, which can satisfy you and also increase metabolism, break down far and at the same time provide the appropriate amount of strength your muscles need. And unfortunately, fast food would do the exact opposite. Fast foods are high in calories and low in Protein, hence why they don't offer any form of satisfaction, yet they lead to weight gain. And to build your muscles, you don't need to be adding calories. Instead, you should burn more than you eat.

Because fast foods are high in the glycemic index, which heightens the body's need for insulin, they provide a mirage rise in the blood sugars, which would fall as quickly as they have risen, prompting hunger.

The automatic response of the body to the increase in insulin production is insulin resistance. And any person who is insulin resistant would overproduce insulin their body isn't using the result in fat burning by increasing fat storage. Insulin resistance reduces the opportunity for the body to send nutrients to the muscles, thereby reducing the prospect of protein synthesis happening

Understand that the result of eating junk and fast food like fries, cheeseburgers, processed meats and sugary snacks put you at a higher risk of putting on pounds. And would pounds and fast food benefit your muscles? No!!!

Junk Foods Builds Dirty Bulking Not Clean Gains

Most junks contain low fibre that is highly palatable. They don't require much chewing and are easily broken down in the mouth. Junks make your palate susceptible to highly stimulating food, in the process reducing your preference for quality, fresh and whole meals. Regular consumption of fast foods breeds an unhealthy diet. A 30g bag of potato chips provides at least 150 calories, out of which 60% calories come from fat, 35% from carbs, and the remaining 5% is gotten from proteins.

Eating junk food would cause you to consume waist-expanding fat, not glute-building Protein. The disadvantage of dirty bulking is that your body would gain fat. Basically, the more you eat junk, the more you store calories as fat rather than being transferred to your muscles,

Even though junk meals and healthy meals calories are derived from a different portion of carbs, fats and proteins in meals, most of the calories gotten from junk would come in the form of fats, processed or refined sugar. While in healthier meals, their calories would be gotten from Protein and carbs rich in fiber.

Junks Offer Empty Calories with No Nutritional Value

Unlike healthy meals, fast food offers an imbalanced proportion of carbs, sugar, Fat and Protein. While most junks might have a marginal amount of Protein, they are largely made up of empty calories. They are regarded as empty calories because they have no real nutritional value.

As per the studies, such a diet is linked to abdominal fat gain, disrupted insulin and glucose homeostasis, and a higher risk of metabolic syndrome. An impaired metabolism makes it harder to build your muscles and contribute to the decrease in energy. When trying to build your gluts and not gain unnecessary fat, getting the right balance of nutrients and calories is essential. And because they are no room for empty calories, you would need to avoid junk foods.

Junks won't Benefit Your Workout or Recovery.

Unlike whole meals, junks don't offer any value to your workouts or recovery. Unfortunately, junks are inexpensive, tasty and convenient fast-food high in sodium, sugar, saturated fats and cholesterol. This highly processed meal is fast food high in calories, low in nutrients, eye-catching, mouthwatering, yet unhealthy. Without a doubt, how much damage and bad impact on your health and muscle building goals the regular eating of junk could cause.

Some of the foods that won't help you achieve your goals of glute growing and muscle gain and should be avoided are:

Alcohol. Alcohol possesses no nutrient at all; they only carry empty calories, and drinking them excessively, can derail your workout sessions the next day.

Processed sugars. Natural sugars from fruits and vegetables help can help keep you charged and fueled for your workouts. Processed sugar, on the other hand, would only increase fat gain.

Fried and processed foods. These kinds of foods are mostly junk, and although they contain some iota of Protein, they are heavy on fats and additives, which can cause an increase can increase to inflammation and support fat gain and not muscle.

The Role Food Plays in Glute Training

Building any muscle in the body would require more than just heavy lifting or working out, even when your goals are increasing strength or hypertrophy. Truthfully the role your diet plays in any time of body composition change, like growing the muscle or losing fat, is as important as the workout routine you indulge in.

Your first decision when you choose to bulk up or grow your glutes might be to go straight into the gym and pick the perfect training session, and that's great, but are you focusing on what you are eating, your macronutrient, calorie intake and the right food to eat and the ones you have to avoid.

Growing your glutes doesn't happen overnight, it is a whole process, but with the right diets, coupled with your training, you would hit you're your strength and hypertrophy goals on time.

Benefits of Food to Muscle Gain

When you are trying to grow a bigger and stronger glute, work out is essential because you would need strength to break down those muscle tissues; from the previous chapter, you would understand the need for muscle breakdown and recovery. During adaption (recovery), those tissues rebuild and become bigger and stronger; however, those new glute muscles don't grow out of anywhere. They grow from the basis of the right nutrient your body has consumed. It is important that to make gains, your body must have the right nutrient to construct muscle.

This means that eating the right food and quantity is essential in growing your glute muscles. Consequently, lifting heavy weights and training without proper nutrition can cause more glute loss than gain, especially without enough Protein.

Inevitably, if you aren't eating right, you wouldn't be charged up with enough strength to workout that would help you grow those glutes muscle.

To get the most gain in muscle growth and strength, you should focus on adding enough calories to your daily meal and enough proteins as protein to help in rebuilding muscle tissue. You must understand the importance of balancing both because if you choose to eat a lot of protein and not enough calories, you will struggle with enough strength for your workout routine to build more glute muscle.

If you eat enough calories and stay heavy on junk and not on enough Protein, you won't be able to grow your glutes. Instead, you would only gain fat.

Quantity of food to Eat When Building Muscle

In the process of growing your glute muscle, your body relies on a lot of food to stay fueled and help in restricting your body composition; this might be a little difficult to accept. Understandably, there is a fear of gaining fat instead of muscles, but those extra calories would go into muscle development and not fat as long as you eat them in the right proportion and training the right way. You might wonder at the appropriate number of calories to consume as an individual per day; your needs per day would vary for each individual. How you work out and gain muscle is unique to each individual. But, adding about 20 to 30 grams of added Protein per day is a good place to start.

Protein (The Building Block for Muscle Growth)

Irrespective of your workout goals, you must ensure you eat a balanced meal. However, you should understand that to focus on growing your glute muscle, getting an adequate protein level is most essential.

During your workout process, your body goes through strenuous exercise, and the more strenuous an exercise is, the more time your muscles would likely need to recover. While paying attention and consistency to your workout, it is important to progress your goals; you should pay attention to your protein diets, which is also important in fostering your progress. Protein, in this case, helps strengthen your body after a workout; this is irrespective of the kind of workout you are doing.

Because your glute tissues are largely made up of Protein, it is important that macronutrients monitored closely. If you are looking bat growing your glutes, you must focus closely on your protein intake and adjust where necessary. Because most western foods are typically rich in Protein, the turnover in inactive people could be slow.

For people looking to add glute muscle mass, here are some general guidelines from research and nutrition organizations that could serve as a guide for your protein consumption:

The American college of sports and academy for nutrition recommend an average amount of 1.2 to 1.7 grams of protein per kilogram of mass for active individuals. This interprets to 95 to 136 grams of protein daily for someone who weighs 150 pounds.

For inactive individuals, about 0.81 grams of protein per kilogram of body mass is enough. This translates to a 120-pound person would eat about 50.5 grams of Protein per day.

The American College of Sports Medicine and the Academy of Nutrition and Dietetics conducted A recent study that analyzed 49 other studies determined that the ideal amount of protein per day for gaining muscle is 1.6

grams per kilogram of body mass. For the 150-pound client, this is 109 grams of protein per day.

Importance of Protein after work out

Proteins are amino acids that serve as your bodies building blocks. This acid is largely responsible for building and repairing the muscle. The Protein we eat breaks down into amino acid which provides the nutrient with your tissues needs for repair and recovery. For clarity, we need protein after a workout to support the healing of our muscles. Because Protein is important to muscle repair, not eating Protein after your workout means that your body would be deprived of nutrients needed for effective and successfully repair. When Protein isn't provided adequately, the muscle tissue won't be able to repair and grow fully, which may lead to inflammation and an increased risk for injury."

Many overuse injuries occur due to insufficient repair nutrients (amino acids from proteins) that the body needs to aid the muscle and tendons and reduce inflammation.

Carbohydrates (the energy block for your muscle growth)

While you are focusing on your protein intake, it is possible to ignore other macronutrients. You must find a balance between the macro and micronutrients. Carbohydrates are energy providers; they are essential to fueling the body for tough workouts that help build muscle. Because the body would struggle to absorb at least 35 grams of nutrients in one sitting, all your meals must contain a balanced share of Protein, carbs and fat. Although fat is considered necessary, it is not important to stay on track with your glute growing. Note that when you consume the appropriate Protein and carbs, you would have enough fat in your diet already. Additionally, fat is easier to store in the body, so it's hard to lack some.

Choosing the right Food for Glute Gain

Fueling your muscle with the right food is important to muscle gains. You'll need lean proteins, foods that are high in protein as well as micronutrients and complex carbohydrates. However, you should understand that knowing what to eat to gain muscle also means avoiding Junk food.

Some of the Best Protein-Rich Foods for glute growing are.

Lean beef. Beef is a good source of protein; this is, of course, when you don't choose lean cuts. In addition to dietary protein benefits, it also contains creatine, which is known for its numerous health benefits and can improve performance during workouts and training.

Cottage cheese. Cottage cheese is known for its calcium benefits, and depending on the type you get, it can provide up 25 grams of protein per portion.

Chicken. Choose chicken breast is a good source of protein, about 26 grams per three ounces.

Beans. Black beans, kidney beans, white beans, and other beans are a great source of lean Protein; they translate into 15 grams per cup. They also contain a load of vitamins, minerals, and fibre.

Greek yoghurt. Yoghurts are a great snack and a key ingredient for smoothies; however, they can be a great supplement for Protein.

Salmon. This fish isn't only rich in fat and omega-3 fatty acids and protein, which is essential to muscle growth.

Quinoa. One cup of this ancient grain includes roughly eight grams of protein and 40 grams of healthy carbohydrates.

Tofu. This meal is made from soybeans; it is an important source of Protein for vegetarians and vegans and is also rich in calcium.

Tuna and Eggs. Tunas are easy to access protein; they could be served as both a meal and a snack. It offers a variety of vitamins and 20 grams of protein in three ounces. Eggs, on the other hand, are rich in both healthy fats and vitamin B. One egg contains six grams of Protein.

Nuts and seeds. Different types of nuts and seeds, including almonds, cashews, walnuts, sunflower seeds, pumpkin seeds, are rich in protein, carbs, and micronutrients

In addition to the protein-rich foods and carbs, like brown rice and beans, it is necessary to fill your day's calories with fruits and vegetables, too, especially before a workout session.

The importance of dark leafy greens

Working out is essential to losing weight and building muscles, but strenuous exercise has a sneaky downside. During the workout, your body releases some oxygen molecule by-products known as free radicals, these radical plays a role in ageing and fosters diseases like diabetes and cancer. No, this doesn't mean you put an end to every form of exercise; just like everything in life, there is always an advantage and disadvantage to things. From the earlier explanation, you would understand the benefit of eating the right foods to your overall health; foods like leafy green vegetables can help reduce the damage associated with strenuous exercise. It could help in minimizing some of the damages to your DNA triggered by free radicals during high-intensity exercise and strenuous exercises.

Together with the numerous vitamins and minerals that green vegetables have to offer, these dark, rich and leafy greens are also rich in compound nitrate. The nitrate content of green veggies is the key to enhancing sporting performance. Similarly, a recent study looked at the potential ergogenic effects of green, leafy vegetables.

These veggies also help strengthen the muscles. Because these leafy greens are packed with nitrates, your body converts these nitrates into nitric oxide.

The role of nitric oxide is to relax the blood and help them widen; this action gives room for the muscles to get a great delivery of oxygen. And because the muscles require more oxygen with the intensity of each exercise, oxygen is essential for creating energy and charging you up as you exercise, which is important for your muscle recovery.

Increased oxygen flow could allow your muscles to perform optimally better, which may ultimately help increase muscle strength and growth.

Pre-Workout and Post Workout

As a fitness enthusiast, you must have people use the phrase pre-workout. A stroll on social media streets would show an average of 43 million people talking about pre-workout. Now, you might wonder what pre-workout are and how relevant they are to your glute training.

What is pre-workout?

Pre work out are supplements claiming to boost training and workout performances when consumed before the exercise. This supplement usually comes in a powder drink mix, but some come in capsules, canned drinks, colorful liquid in bottles, and chews with the promise of bettering your workout performance.

Although there is no good definition of what a pre work out is. Generally, you can describe it as a formula or production to boost the energy level of athletes through the combination of proposed antioxidants, vitamins, and carbs.

It is important to understand that no two supplements are the same or even similar in ingredients despite the numerous supplement products out there. Some pre-workouts may contain carbs; those carbs are usually calorie-free, while others may contain caffeine, an amino acid that would end up increasing blood flow to your muscles at the same time dilating your blood vessels.

Some pre-workout supplements may contain the esoteric ingredient, which increases your degree of insulin growth factor; this hormone is what your body should naturally produce in response to resistance training to foster tissue and muscle growth.

Most people result in taking pre-workout supplements are majorly for performance reasons and to feel fueled up when working out.

However, if your goal is to grow your glutes, pre-workout supplements have no direct impact on their growth. But, if you are comfortable with taking them after doing your due diligence in research, then you can. You may be curious if these supplements practice what they preach?

It's a mixed bag: Some pre-workout ingredients are well-studied and can help improve your performance but may probably not; if you can weight train without the need for a supplement, then you don't need it.

Post Workout

Working out or training is a beneficial yet strenuous and complex activity. During your workout, the exercise isn't the only aspect where you pay all of your attention. You should understand that what you do after your workout is also important for your optimal health and effectiveness.

Stretching after workouts

Having enough body flexibility is as important as your strength and endurance training; why is this important?

Stretching helps you build a healthy range of muscle motion around your joints; stretching should be done regularly; some of the benefits are:

- It increases efficiency during a workout.
- It lowers the risks of musculoskeletal system injury during exercise and in your daily activity.
- It helps decrease stress during muscle training, and aides' post-workout tension relief
- Improves body posture caused by the extension of certain target muscle groups.

The optimal time for stretching is always at the end of your workout because it is at this time that your muscles are warmed up and relaxed. They have attained maximum elasticity. In addition to stretching after your workout, your post-workout meal is as important in beating your goals. As discussed above, you understand the body's most preferred power source during exercise is glycogen deposited by carbohydrates into the liver and muscle. When you don't top up your tank with carbohydrates to give you energy, you begin to feel irritable, exhausted, and an acute pang of hunger, which can invariably lead to binge eating.

Hence, why a moderate size carbohydrate snack must be an excellent choice? Because during a workout session, you are destroying the muscles to regrow them and change their quality. Because muscles are built from Protein, a meal rich in protein can boost the process of muscle growth and recovery. Consequently, the best food to eat after a workout would be a carbohydrate snack with a combination of Protein.

For pre work out and post work out nutrition, you would understand that it is all about your timing, Protein and carb intake, irrespective of your dietary preference.

Because you aim to add glute mass, you must eat before and after your workout; however, if your workout isn't more than an hour and it's an early morning cardio session, you might not need to eat before you begin. But if it is a prolonged training session, you would find it beneficial to have a small snack before the session begins. Protein and carbohydrates are highly essential to post-workout and should be consumed within an hour post-workout

For a vegan diet, Protein is found in a lot of plant-based foods, some of which are:

- Lentils and beans
- Tempeh, tofu, edamame and soy products
- Seeds
- Whole grains
- Nuts

Vegans are to ensure they are conscious and deliberate about their protein intake. If you are unsure that you're not hitting your protein requirements, it would be beneficial to consult a dietitian.

Ten vegan pre-workout snacks

Soymilk Fruit smoothie

Low-fat muesli with soy

Coconut yoghurt

Grapes, mango and banana

Slices of whole grain with peanut butter and banana slices

Banana ice cream prepared from a blend of frozen banana and plant milk

Cup of soy milk/soy yoghurt

Boiled sweet potato/potato

Overnight oats prepared with almond or soy milk

Soy-cheese sandwich and salad

Ten vegan post-workout snacks and meals

Fruit smoothie with soy or nut milk and a few scoops of soy or coconut yoghurt

Slice of whole-grain toast or crackers with peanut butter

A pack of nuts and fresh or dried fruit or bliss balls

Vegetable ginger-soy stir-fry soup with tofu and basmati rice

Medium size of baked beans, other beans you prefer

Spaghetti Bolognese made with lentil

Salad made with hummus and tabbouleh, and a cup of soy milk

Rolled oats topped with soy yoghurt, chopped nuts, chia seeds, and any berry of your choice

Lentil burger with salad on a multi-grain bun

Baked beans on toast with mushroom and roasted tomato

A good diet makes you healthy and gives you the booty of your dreams. You can also grow your glutes with the right diet. Not all the meals you eat are good for your body. You already know that. It's time for you to follow the diet in this chapter so you can attain your booty goals in no time.

CHAPTER 7
SHEDDING FAT WITHOUT LOSING GLUTE GAIN

You might have added fat in the process of gaining glute, and that's ok. However, just because you want to shed some fat doesn't mean you should shed some hard gain muscles, should you? Some would argue that losing fat while maintaining glute muscles is an impossible goal, as those two goals are contrasting. Others believe it is only possible through surgical methods and not through fitness, but with the proper mindset and fitness plan, it is definitely possible.

When your goal is to shed some fat but maintain your glute muscle, you would need to cut down on some calorie intake. Cutting down on your calorie intake would mean that the size of your glute and muscle gain would also decrease, but it could be replenished by implementing HIIT exercise. HIIT exercise is a form of training targeted at rebuilding specific muscles, in this case, your glutes. Understand that no two person's butts are the same, so most often, your result despite the exercise may largely depend on your genetic make-up and body's physique. Also, note that numerous diets and exercises are known to help you supposedly lose weight and maintain your glute mass. A number of these diets and exercises don't do the justice you require. Check out this complied and comprehensive knowledge to guide you on your journey to a leaner yet muscular body.

What is HIIT Training?

Irrespective of your workout or training type, chances are high that at some point, you have heard of the term HIIT which stands for high-intensity training. But what then is HIIT, and how can it be beneficial to shedding fat while maintaining glute?

What is HIIT?

Possibly, you might have an idea of what HIIT means, but like many workout routines in the fitness world, there are many misconceptions attached to what HIIT truly is, how you can make the most of them and how to teach them into your workout session.

Here's what you need to know about this popular training method.

You would understand that HIIT refers to a particular type of training from the name high-intensity interval training. However, you should note that it is possible to carry out interval training without involving in any HIIT workout or routine. The prerequisite for HIITS workout is being repeated, basically repeating tough sets of workouts with interspersed and a period reserved for recovery or rest. The hallmark of this exercise is how during your intervals, you'll be challenging yourself nearly to your max.

The HIIT is the exact opposite of going for a long stretch of exercise where the rationale behind it is to conserve your energy while you sustain the activity for much longer. For instance, going on a long easy run. Basically, HIIT means a short fragment of intense exercise carried out at short intervals that take turns with a lower degree of the recovery period. It can also be referred to as one of the most effective ways of exercising.

Typically, most HIIT workouts will range from 5 to 30 minutes in duration, but it can produce twice as many health benefits as the normal degree exercise despite the short duration of this workout. During HIIT exercise, recovery before your next set of reps is vital. Aligning your body to get accustomed to two very distinct consistently would provide excellent cardio transformation. The rest period is needed to get the body in tune and prepare it to perform at its best during the intense workout. The main activity performed during HIIT varies but can be sprinting, high knees, burpee, biking, press up, jump rope and various bodyweight exercises. For instance, during a HIIT workout, a high knee could be carried out for about 20 to 30 seconds of exercise as fast as possible against high resistance; this would be closely followed by several minutes of slow, easy movement with low resistance for about 10 seconds.

This series of activities would be considered one "round" or "rep" of HIIT, and you would be required to complete 4 to 6 reps or rounds in one workout. However, you should note that the amount of time required for each rep and recovery time would be based on the intensity and the type of exercise you have chosen.

Regardless of how it is performed, high-intensity intervals should contain short periods of severe activity that make your heart rate accelerate up. Not only have that, HIIT delivered the benefits of longer-duration exercise in a much shorter length of time while providing some unique health benefits.

Benefits of HIIT

Although many people are familiar with the positive effect of this activity, it is estimated that an average of 30% of people worldwide doesn't get enough of it.

People who have a physically demanding job should find a dedicated fitness routine in other to stay active. Unfortunately, many feel that they don't have enough time to exercise. If this is you, maybe you should try high-intensity interval training (HIIT)? Alternatively, if your goal is to lose weight efficiently, try HIIT exercises.

One of the most significant advantages of HIIT is that you can get maximal health benefits in a minimal time. Read on to find the top 7 health benefits of HIIT workouts.

1. **HIIT Helps Burn More Calories**

Your body burns the same number of calories during your HIIT workout, the same as what it would burn during your typical workout routine like skipping and running. Bear in mind that the HIIT workout is usually shorter. However, the benefit of HIIT is, your body burns more calories after the workout with HIIT workout than during a regular exercise where your heart is relatively stable. After your regular workout, your heart finds its rhythm and is relatively stable, but for HIIT, more calories are burned even after the exercises. Studies have shown that an average of 3 kilocalories is burned per minute during HIIT, compared to 2.8 kilocalories burned during regular exercise. The idea of calories burning after you have stopped exercising is a process called post-exercise oxygen consumption (EPOC).

EPOC happens when your body burns more calories during the process of healing the wear and tear you get from an intense workout. This happens because the HIIT exercises are intense in nature; consequently, EPOC has been associated with effective muscle growth.

2. HIIT is Ideal for Weight Loss

As a result of EPOC, HIIT burns more calories than the traditional form of exercise. It can also be a more convenient way to burn more calories and lose weight since you won't spend so much time on work out. Basically, HIIT would stir up your rate, which is optimal for shedding calories and the most effective way to lose weight. As a result of its effective way to lose weight, HIIT has become a popular workout in the fitness world. When you want to shed some fat, at the same time retain and build lean muscles to continue to burn more fat, HIIT is the best option for you. This is because it forces your body to break down fat while deriving energy from them as opposed to carbohydrates, which makes losing fat more effective.

In contrast, being on a diet would make it difficult to lose fat while maintaining muscle. But research has shown that with HIIT, you can preserve those hard-earned muscles while burning the maximum amount of fat.

In 2019 a study was conducted by the British Journal of Sports Medicine, where 77 studies were analyzed. The result showed revealed that people who partook in HIIT workouts lost 28.5% more fat than people who participated in the moderately-intense exercise, like jumping.

The study surveyed the effect of HIIT on some 46 men who were overweight. These participants, who were on the average age of 25 years, participated in 3, 20 minutes HIIT workout sessions a week. After 12 weeks, those in the HIIT exercise group had obtained a greater decrease in abdominal fat compared to those in the other group.

However, the added advantage to the HIIT exercise is it the effect of all the intense workout that keeps your body in a prolonged state of fat shedding, long after your exercise. This means your body would be burning fat up to 24 hours after the workout.

3. HIIT increases Metabolic Rate and improve heart health

One major benefit of HIIT workout is its ability to burn calories even after the exercise has been completed. There are numerous studies to back up the demonstrated and tremendous benefit of HIIT exercise to increase metabolism. Some studies have even shown that HIIT increases metabolism after exercise more than running or even weight training. In a similar study, HIIT was also found to transfer the body's metabolism regarding using fat for energy instead of a carb.

While another study revealed that an average of 2 minutes of HIIT exercise in the form of sprinting is capable of increasing metabolism for over 24 hours which is as much as 35 minutes of running, as well as its benefit to increase in fat shedding and muscle retention, HIIT exercise serves as a form stimulation to the production of HGH human growth hormones. The hormones go up by 450% during the 24 hours following your workout. This would typically increase your metabolism in the short term, however with consistency in HIIT workouts, and your overall metabolism rate would experience a surge. The increase and improvement in the rate of metabolism would make it almost impossible to gain weight. Also, an improved and healthy metabolism would aid your system in getting rid of toxins and improve your body's efficiency. While HIIT exercise could help in improving metabolic health, it also improves heart health in people with good health conditions, alongside those with cardiovascular conditions, blood pressure, blood sugar levels, and cholesterol, and as mentioned above, it could help burn calories even after your HIIT workout is done. Improving your cardiovascular health is perhaps one of the most important benefits of HIIT exercise. This is because people would generally not want to push themselves into the anaerobic zone. HIIT exercise generally provides the benefit of getting you there within a short time with a dash of resting time to provide strength to your heart and consume oxygen.

With the increase in heart disease, one-quarter of the deaths in the US are heart disease-related. Improving the state of cardiovascular health can reduce the risk of heart disease, making HIIT workouts a great investment.

4. HIIT can build muscle groups

A number of HIIT workout involves a different kind of movement. These movements allow your body to work out a different group of muscles at the same time. For instance, a HIIT workout might have you do high knees, squats, burpees, and push-ups, focusing on different muscle groups. The HIIT workout's intensity would help strengthen and improve your muscles' ability to keep working out. The HIIT also training boosts muscular endurance because the muscles do not get enough rest.

In addition, during a study in 2017 in Diabetology & Metabolic Syndrome, results showed that a 12 minutes HIIT workout would have more effect on the muscles than a 45 minutes' workout session of aerobic workout amongst overweight female teens. The tool of measurement for this study was tracking the level of irisin, a hormone expelled by the muscles as a response to exercise. Asides from the fat burning, and preserved and improved muscles, HIIT exercise also increases the human growth hormone. The human growth hormone (HGH) is not just responsible for the heightened burning of calories and fat, but it also slows down the process of ageing, which is another sneaky benefit of the HIIT exercise. Consequently, if you feel a decline in your weight loss journey or your journey to fitness has plummeted, consider investing in HIIT workouts.

5. HIIT Improves Oxygen Consumption

The human heart pumps blood from the circulatory system in order to deliver oxygen and nutrients to your muscles. And research has shown numerous evidence that HIIT workouts can support and even strengthen your circulatory system.

Your muscle's ability to utilize oxygen is referred to as oxygen consumption. Endurance training is typically how your body improves on your oxygen's consumption. Generally, this would consist of prolonged sessions of continuous moderate exercises like running or skipping at a steady rate. However, studies have shown that HIIT exercise c produce the same benefits and result in a shorter time frame. This study further proves that five weeks of HIIT training performed 20 minutes for each rep 4 days a week could improve oxygen consumption by 9%. This result was similar to another study which showed that cycling continuously for an average of 40 minutes per day, four times a week.

6. It is Efficient

If you operate on a busy schedule, then HIIT is the right exercise for you. Whether you want to squeeze in a quick workout session between work and kids drop off, HIIT is typically the ideal workout for a busy lifestyle because it can be done anywhere. The average time for a HIIT session is around 25 to 30 minutes. However, there are a number of HIIT workouts that last as little as 4 minutes. Studies have shown that progress can be achieved from a 15 minutes HIIT workout session at least 4 times a week than jogging on a treadmill for an hour daily.

If you want to quickly have a workout session or jump in and out of the gym, HIIT is your best option. And according to a 2011 study presented at the American College of Sports Medicine Annual Meeting, "two weeks of high-intensity intervals is synonymous to six to eight weeks of endurance training when improving your aerobic capacity". Basically, a HIIT workout is one of the most effective ways of getting your heart rate up.

7. Do It from Anywhere

Not only are HIIT efficient, but they involve series of short, intense ranges of different aerobic exercises. Running, jump roping, biking fits into that category. High knees, squat, jump the twist, jumping jacks or jumping rope, burpee, press up, and thrust are some of the activities that fit into this category. HIIT are basically plyometric work that allows your heart rate to build up your endurance.

One of the most interesting factors associated with HIITS is that they don't require any equipment or technical training for an effective workout.

Since the idea of HIIT is to engage in maximum-intensity exercises for a short period and then recover for an even shorter period, you can adjust it to fit any time and space constraints and still get all the benefits!

Strangely, some equipment like dumbbells can make HIIT less effective. This is because you want the focus on pushing your heart to its max, not your biceps. Here are a few no-equipment workouts to get you started on HIIT.

HIIT Exercise for Beginners

For beginners who are looking to start a HIIT workout, there are a few details you must have in mind about the kind of exercise before you get started.

From the above discussion, you would understand what the HIIT exercise is. High-intensity interval training is a form of workout that spreads across a short series but intense hard work with easier recovery periods. Although there is no set formula for the HIIT exercise, the workouts require that they be kept short with a set time for a rest period in other to reach maximal capacity for your desired goal.

To get you started, you should understand that the real HIIT is quite different from the general understanding of most exercisers and even fitness enthusiasts you see in most fitness classes. With the correct HIIT, you go all out for 20 to 30 seconds to connect with your aerobic system to provide you energy, while your rest would be half as long.

For one, because you are relatively new to this exercise, you must pay attention to the moves and how it is down. With HIIT, it is always quality over quantity or speed, so don't give up form in exchange for more reps and speed during execution. This is because you will be pushing your effort level higher than you are comfortable with. And you would be doing straight reps and sets of an exercise, so you'll be increasing your heart rate and essentially gaining cardiovascular benefits.

Also, beginners should ensure they feel comfortable with the movements before trying to do them. Unless you are comfortable with a set number of reps required during a HIIT exercise, don't be tempted into jumping into more activity than you would averagely do. You should also pay attention to your pain, ensure to listen to your body and focus on the pain around your joints. They might feel different from the muscle tension you would feel during regular exercise. Note that when you begin to feel pain or discomfort more than the average level, you should stop. And if you acquire any injury during the course of your HIIT exercise, please ensure you speak with a doctor or therapist immediately. Ensure that you have fully recovered before starting any exercise program.

It is important to build on your form to make sure you can do an exercise with proper form at an easy tempo before kicking it up to high intensity.

Warm-ups are also crucial to HIIT exercise, irrespective of if your exercise would be cardio based HIIT or strength HIIT. The intensity of HIIT exercises increases the more you work out, hence why it is important to warm up your body. Warm-ups are more like prepping your body and nervous system for work. Your warm-up should include Some mobility moves, like hip-opening stretches and thoracic spine rotations. Without warming up, your body isn't ready to work, making it susceptible to poor performance or injury. Typically, the higher the intensity of your workout, the more important the warm-up is and required.

From the previous chapter, you would have a proper understanding of why you should eat before your workout. It is no different for HIIT, HIIT is one challenging workout, and in other to go hard, your body would need energy. This can be really difficult when your body doesn't have a sufficient supply of carbs.

Continuous cardio steady burns and can be done on an empty stomach even though it is not advisable, but with HIIT, there would be a decrease in performance if you try working out on an empty stomach. Not only would your body struggle with performance, you would most likely find yourself going off balance and scramble for energy as the intensity of your exercise hit, but your body has nothing to grab.

Hence, the essence of having a healthy snack or meal before your HIIT workout, because without enough carbs, your body would struggle.

One major mistake you should be mindful of as a beginner is scheduling a long HIIT session. Instead, it is advisable you split your workout session with rest in between, rather than going a full 45 or 30 minutes before resting. And in all that, you do not underestimate the power of rest and recovery. Ensure you prioritize frequent rest in between intense workouts; neglecting your rest days can not only lead to diminishing performance returns, but it can also leave you open to injury, fatigue, or burnout. Make sure you're balancing them with plenty of easy workouts—as well as at least one straight recovery day per week.

Without a doubt, intervals during your HIIT are important, but what happens you're your intervals becomes too long? Any HIIT interval that lasts longer than 30 seconds is having a reverse effect on your goals. It is important to stay within your range of 15- to 30-second, don't overstretch it. The objective of HIIT exercise is to go as fast and hard as possible during your workout, and you would only have a small window of time to achieve that before fatigue sets in.

As a beginner, don't make the mistake of overdoing your HIIT exercise. There is a popular misconception that more is better. However, this often leads to burnout, injury and fatigue. With HIIT, consistency is important, but your body only needs three to five days of workout per workout. Good sleep, stretching and healthy eating are also important.

For an efficient 20 – 30-minute HIIT workout for beginners, here's how to get started.

The Workout

Requirement: An exercise mat for ease and a pair of sliders. (If there are no sliders, a paper towel will do just fine)

Exercises

set 1

Push-up

Reverse lunge

set 2

Side shuffle with floor tap

Slider arm circles

STEPS

Complete 20 seconds of backward lunges and 10 seconds of push-ups for set 1. Repeat. Take a minute to relax. Finish all five rounds.

Complete each exercise for 30 seconds in set 2. (Switch sides halfway through for the arm circles). Take a minute to relax. Finish all five rounds.

For beginners, you might not be comfortable go for all five-round, and that's ok. If you may feel more comfortable completing two or three rounds of each superset.

Directions

Push-up

Start with your palms flat, hands shoulder-width apart, shoulders stacked directly above your wrists, legs extended behind you, and core and glutes engaged in a high plank.

Lower your chest to the floor by bending your elbows.

Straighten your arms by pushing through the palms of your hands. This is one repetition. Complete for a total of 10 seconds.

Reverse Lunge

With your feet shoulder-width apart and your core engaged, then stand.

To sink into a lunge, step back with your right foot and bend both knees. Maintain a strong core, tucked hips, and a straight back.

Push off your right foot and take a step forward to get back to your starting position.

Rep on the opposite side. For a total of 20 seconds, alternate sides.

The reverse lunge builds your quadriceps and your glutes.

Push-ups, which engage your chest, shoulders, and core muscles, can be a difficult form for beginners; you might feel more at ease modifying by using an incline for balance and support. The easier the move will be, the higher the step or box. Elevating your hands instead of lowering your knees is a more efficient approach to make push-ups easier because it helps you retain tension and stability throughout your core and the rest of your body, rather than breaking at the knees. This will make it easier for you to move to a full push-up.

Side Shuffle with Floor Tap

Clasp your hands at chest height, with your feet hip-width apart as you stand, core engaged.

Begin by bending your knees slightly and sending your butt back into a half squat.

Shuffle as swiftly as possible to the right for four to five feet from that position (or as space allows). Move your feet quickly, concentrating on speed more than the size of each stride.

Tap the floor with your right hand when you reach the end.

Shuffle to the left and tap the floor with your left hand.

For 30 seconds, keep moving back and forth as swiftly as possible

As beginners, you can keep this low workout impact by keeping this workout by removing the shuffle, making lateral lunges instead, and skipping the floor tap if it feels uncomfortable for your back.

Slider Arm Circles

Begin with a high plank, with your hands shoulder-width apart, shoulders over the wrist put a glider under each hand. Straighten your core and engage your glutes

Clasp your land hand unto a slider, and slow imitate a counterclockwise circle. You could reverse the movement to draw a clockwise circle for each rep. Tighten your core and glutes and try not to let your hips move.

Do this for 15 seconds, then switch sides.

The slider arm circles exercise gives your core muscles and your shoulder stability.

Beginner HIIT Workouts that Can Do in 30 Minutes or Less

10-Minute HIIT Workout

In less than ten minutes, you could work up a HIIT workout session with no equipment, right in the comfort of your home or wherever you want

3 rounds 20 seconds and 10 seconds' rest

Jab, cross, front (left)

Jumping jacks

Sumo squats

Jab, cross, front (right)

Direction

Jab, cross, front (right side): as you stand, ensure your right foot are in front of your left. With your hips facing your left side, put your arms up into boxing like position.

Throw a punch forward with the right arm, then throw a "cross" punch with the left arm, allowing your body to rotate as your left arm interchanges over your body to the right. Your body weight should rest over your right foot, with the back of your heel slightly picking off the floor. Place both arms back into the body, then shift your weight back to the starting position as you face front. Repeat on the left side.

Jumping jacks: Start by standing straight with your feet hip-width apart and your arms resting at your sides. Jump up with your feet out while raising your arms. Repeat as fast as possible. If regular jumping jacks are too difficult, try stepping side to side as you raise your arms instead.

Sumo squats: Place your feet apart more than your hip width. Point your toes out at 40 degrees. Balancing your weight on your heels, your back flat, and your chest up, lower your body until your thighs are side by side to the floor.

Thoroughly engage your glutes and quads and move back to the start position, then repeat.

Cool down with an overhead stretch, forward fold and reverse lung.

20-Minute HIIT Workout

This is a form of HIIT Metabolic conditioning workout designed to capitalize on your caloric burn. The HIIT metabolic conditioning can be a little challenging because it is more intense than your regular HIIT workout. Your body can go through five moves that focus on full-body exercises. Try to complete as many reps as possible during each 45-second interval, then rest for 15 seconds before repeating.

3 rounds, 45 seconds, 15 seconds' rest.

Push-ups

Tricep dips

Butt kicks

Side lunges

Squats

Directions

Push-ups: If a traditional push up is difficult for you, try supporting yourself by placing your hands on a well-balanced chair or table instead of the floor. Or you could try doing a push up with your knees resting on the ground.

Squats: For added support, use a chair for assistance. Ensure you keep your feet under your hips and your bodyweight resting on your heels for maximum result.

Butt kicks: you could either jog or walk in a place while you kick your right heel up to touch your bottom. do the same with your left leg.

Tricep dips: Hold your back to the chair or position your hands on a chair or a low table. Put your legs straight out in front of you and balance on your palms. Lower yourself as far as you can by bending your elbows, then press back up to the starting position. Activate your core!

Side Lunges: your toes facing forwards and your bodyweight resting on your heels and, step to the left in a lateral lunge, placing your knee above your toes. Alternate between your legs.

Cool down with an overhead stretch, a forward fold and a quad stretch.

30-Minute HIIT Workout

If you have got half an hour to spare, you could try a longer workout to challenge your core, upper body and lower body strength. If you are a beginner with no prior experience, it is advisable to stick with the 10 and 20 minutes HIIT workout. Additionally, this workout is known to burn more calories than 30 minutes spent walking on a treadmill.

3 rounds 45 seconds, 15 seconds' rest

Push up

Squats

Butt kicks

Tricep dips

Side lunges

Jumping jacks

Sit-ups

Try This 20-Minute HIIT Workout for Your Butt

This HIIT workout is effective for your glute, can be done anywhere, at any time and would give your butt a good lift while burning calories and increasing metabolism. Considering you would be getting thorough value for just 20 to 30 minutes, there's no reason to skip these exercises; you could even do them in between meetings or your lunch break. The workout specifically targets all 3 parts of your butt (gluteus maximus, gluteus medius and gluteus minimus).

90 seconds of walking lunges

30 seconds of squats

90 seconds of curtsy lunges

30 seconds of squat jumps

30 seconds of squat jumps

1-minute donkey kicks (right)

1-minute donkey kicks (left)

30 seconds of squats

1 minute of fire hydrants

30 seconds of single-leg glute bridge (right)

30 seconds of single-leg Glute Bridge (left)

Rest until your time is at 15 minutes

Repeat twice

From our previous chapter, you would understand the benefit of stretching to your body; stretching can also be applied for HIIT exercise, especially as a beginner. Your body is put under a lot of pressure during HIIT training, and in a bid to lose rigid knots and improve mobility, consider holding a stretch for about 30-40 seconds, it could be longer if you desire after each session.

Lastly, because you are new to the ropes of HIIT exercise, begin with a more full-body workout rather than focusing on exercise targeted to a specific body area or muscle group (like the HIIT glute workout). This is not to stop you from growing glutes. However, it is to ensure you don't run the risk of injury. Focusing intense workouts on one area can increase the risk of injury since you are still learning to build a strong strength base.

Combined Interval HIIT Workout

If you want to try different intervals in one session, you can try this killer HIIT routine that you can knock some sweat out of you out in less than 15 minutes.

Burpees for 30 seconds. Rest for 15 seconds.

Squat jumps for 45 seconds. Rest for 15 seconds.

V-ups for 30 seconds. Rest for 15 seconds.

Downward dog ankle reaches for 45 seconds. Rest for 15 seconds.

Do burpees for 30 seconds. Rest for 15 seconds.

Repeat twice.

Tabata-Style HIIT Workout

Tabata-style HIIT is easy to follow yet super challenging workout. Traditionally a Tabata workout features up to eight sets of 20 seconds on and 10 seconds off for a total of four minutes.

However, you can choose to apply the timing to your activity of choice or switch up the quantity to 45 seconds on, 15 seconds off. Try this bodyweight Tabata sequence below to get your heart pounding and mix and match exercises based on your ability level and preferences.

Air squats for 20 seconds. Then rest for 10 seconds.

Mountain climbers for 20 seconds. Then rest for 10 seconds.

Do lunges for 20 seconds, alternating legs as you go. Then rest for 10 seconds.

Do burpees for 20 seconds. Then rest for 10 seconds.

Repeat three more times.

With all of these, when implemented properly, you can be assured that you can shed stubborn fat without losing your hard-earned gained glute muscle.

CHAPTER 8

GLUTE STRETCHES

Your Glute is one of the most important muscles in your body; they work hard and play a crucial role in many functional and locomotive movements. Your glutes help you with any task you might consider mundane, like climbing, standing, walking, climbing stairs, and standing up from a chair. They are attached to bones in your hips, back, pelvis, back, and waist, and are located in your butt area, and are considered the largest muscle group in the body. Hence, the reason why when your glutes are tight, you might feel the tension in major parts of your body like your buttocks, hips, back, waist, and other surrounding areas. With the number of functions your glute muscle performs, it is important to activate the glutes every day during your warm-up and to do glute stretches during and after completing your workouts.

A lot of people experience muscle tightness after staying inactive for a long time, and it could also happen when you strain or overwork your muscles during a workout or during athletic activities. Here, we'll explain the process of starching your glutes, how-to, and the benefits.

Also, living a sedentary lifestyle and overuse from running too much can both lead to tight glutes. Tighten glutes would cause a muscular imbalance in your kinetic chain, which can lead to injury, lower back pain, issues with your IT band, runner's knee, and piriformis.

It is common to experience delayed onset muscle soreness or muscle tightness (DOMS) when you start working out. This is because your muscles are beginning to adapt to flexibility and are utilized in different ways.

Consequently, if you don't treat your cheeks right, your performance would be affected. All your glutes would require from you is a little TLC and stretching regularly, this is irrespective if you are not active, or your mileage is high. All you need to do is to start incorporating these Glute stretches into your daily routine to ensure you keep running your butt off, injury-free.

Delayed Onset Muscle Soreness (DOMS)

The pain you experience in your muscles after you work out is known as delayed onset muscle soreness (DOMS). Typically, you would experience DOMS a day or two after your workout; you won't feel DOMS at the time of the workout. In contrast, the pain felt during or immediately after your workout session is a different form of muscle soreness, which is known as acute muscle soreness (AMS).

Acute muscle soreness is caused by the quick buildup of lactic acid. It is that burning sensation you would feel in your muscle during your workout or immediately after exercising. However, the pain often disappears as fast as they build up or a short period after your exercise.

How to Spot DOMS?

Research from the American College of sports medicine has shown that DOMS symptoms averagely occur at least 12 to 24 hours after a workout. It's natural to experience a peak in about one to three days after your workout and relief after that.

Symptoms of DOMS may include:

- fatigue in the muscle
- short-term loss of muscular strength
- sensitive and tender to touch muscles
- Decrease in range of motion caused by pain and stiffness with each movement
- swelling in the affected muscles

What causes DOMS?

Delayed onset muscles can be caused by high-intensity exercise. They cause tiny and microscopic tears to your muscle's fiber. Your body's response to this damage is to increase inflammation, which invariably would lead to delayed onset of soreness in the muscles.

Basically, any high-intensity exercise can cause DOMS, but a particular type is known as eccentric exercise, often triggers it.

Eccentric exercises cause you to tense a muscle while you lengthen it.

Who Can Experience DOMS?

DOMS can affect just about anyone, from elite athletes to beginners, to people who haven't worked out in a long time. So, DOMS is no respecter of your fitness level. It can strike whether you dial up your workout intensity, partake in eccentric exercises, or try a new kind of exercise your body isn't familiar with.

What are the benefits of stretching your glutes?

When your glutes begin to feel tightened, stretching them is the perfect way you can relieve tension. You could also relieve pressure and discomfort like:

- Pelvic pain
- Buttocks pain
- Tight hips
- Pain in your hips
- Lower back pain
- Pain in the knee
- Tightened hamstrings

Additionally, by relieving tension, glute stretches may help you

- enhance your flexibility even till old age
- increases and build your range of motion
- decreases your risk of injury

- strengthens and improve your mobility
- Decreases your chances of having accidental injuries, especially injury in your knees
- Relieves the stiffness you feel after working out. (Glutes stretches are beneficial after a workout too)
- Improves your body posture.
- Reduces and delays fatigue on the glute muscles.
- Increases your athletic performance.
- Helps break down body fat.

At What point should you stretch your glutes?

The important fact about glute stretches is that they can be done as part of your warm-up before your exercise and after your workout. Stretching your glutes before your exercise can get your blood flowing to your targeted muscles in preparation for the movement and activity. Glute stretches are also important after your workout because they can foster flexibility, and put a stop to stiffness, and at the same time boost your overall performance when next you work out.

However, you can always stretch your glutes if you have been inactive or if they feel tightened as you go about your daily activities like when you splurge, watch your favorite TV show, or are sitting at your desk for hours.

Here is several Glute stretches to help you relax your glutes, as well as your back, legs, hips, and pelvis.

Stretching Your Glutes before a Workout

It is important that you partake in warm-ups before your workout so as to ensure your body is prepared for the exercise and to also reduce the risk of injury. Warm-ups are generally dynamic stretches that help improve blood flow and increase your range of motion towards the target area.

Here are some ways you can stretch and warm up your glutes before starting your workout session:

Foam rolling

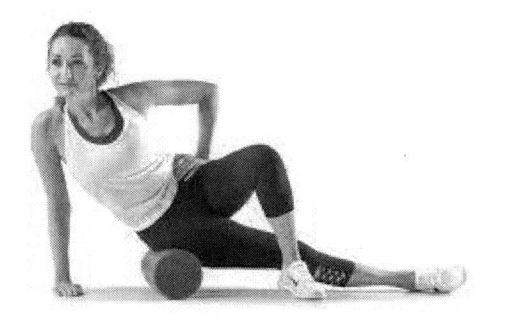

Proform.com

Foam rolling is a dynamic exercise that is often used as part of muscle recovery exercise. However, it can also double as a form of glute stretch workout before your workout. It helps to warm up the glutes by increasing blood flow to the Glute and unravel connecting tissues around the glute muscle to ensure there is seamless and smooth movement.

Directions

- Horizontally Place the foam roller behind you and sit carefully on top of the roller foam as you place both hands face down on the floor behind you.

- Raise and turn out your left leg to ensure that your ankle is resting on your left just above your knees, as shown in the image above.

- Gently turn your hips to the left to give room for the foam roller to have direct contact and press into your right Glute.

- Gradually roll the foam across the length of your gluteal. Once you get to a soft or tender spot (a trigger point), pause and stay in that position for at least 50 seconds or when you feel the pain or tenderness has reduced tremendously. You can also choose to perform little strokes over tender spots if you choose.

- Roll down the foam across the length of your Glute continuously and slow down when you get to the trigger point.

Repeat on the right side.

Leg Swings

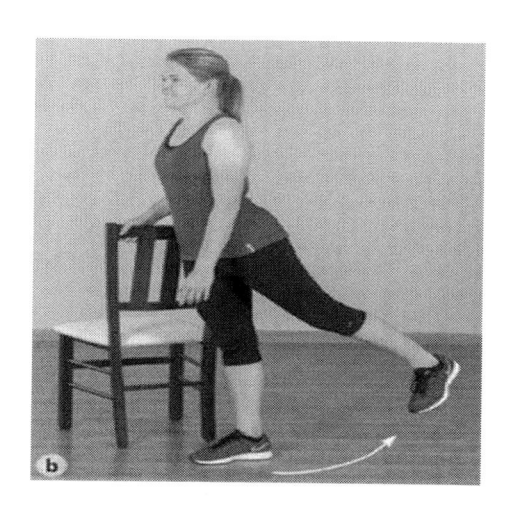

Leg swing is an effective way to warm up your hips and glutes. You can do them before a workout or as a means to warm up your muscles before deep stretching.

Directions

- Place both your hands at the back of a chair. With your hands resting on the chair, position both feet on the floor, hip-width apart.

- As you keep your left foot firmly on the floor. Keep your right legs straight and swing them back to your body. Ensure that your torso remains erect as you do this.

- While your torso remains upright, swing your right leg forward, directly in front of your body.

- Continuously swing your leg forward and backward before switching sides.

Lateral Banded Walk

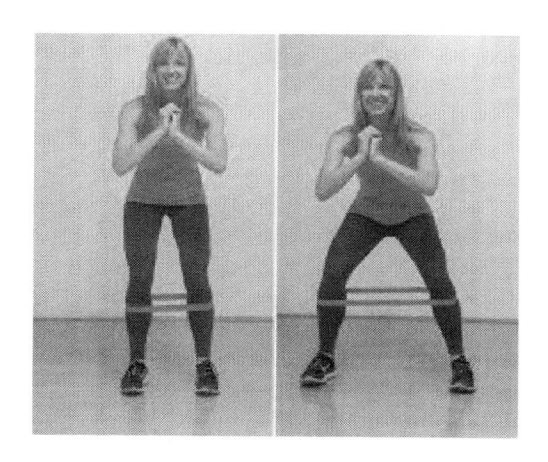

Popsugar.com

The lateral walk improves balance during the exercise and prevents muscular injury. It fully engages the glutes, thighs, and hips. The lateral walk also strengthens major glute muscles.

Directions

- With a resistance band hooked to your ankles, place booth feet hip wide apart on the floor. Do well to keep the knee in line with your toes as you stand upright. This would be your starting position.

- With your right foot on the floor, place your left foot forward to ensure that your feet are a little bit farther than a wide hip distance.

- With your left foot still positioned on the floor, move your right foot inwards to go back to your starting position.

- Keeping your left foot on the floor, step your right foot inwards to return to the starting position.

Repeat the process, but ensure you complete the same number of reps on each side.

Single-leg Romanian deadlift & knee hug

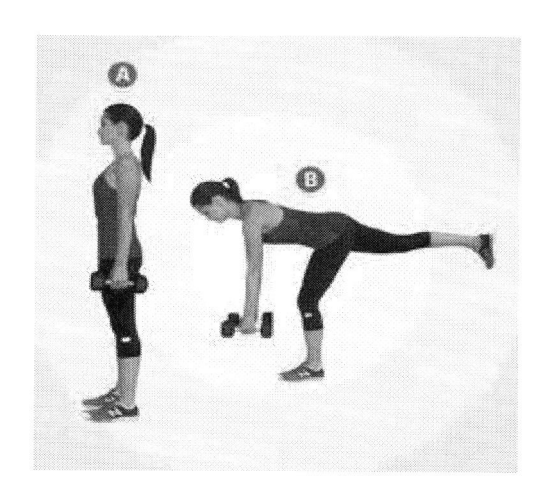

Skimble.com

Any muscle used for balance (especially the Glute) would be strengthened by the single-leg Romanian deadlift. It functions as a unilateral exercise, so it can help you enhance the balance between your legs.

Directions

To start, firmly place your right foot on the ground and release your left leg, then bring your right knee up into your chest area.

Slightly bend your right knees and set this position at a fixed angle. Without changing the angle of your right knees, bend forward until your upper body is facing the floor while extending your left leg behind you. Extend your arms to the floor as you do this. Make sure that you maintain your hips level and keep a high chest with your head as an extension of your spine. You should feel tension at the back of your right leg (your hamstring).

Using your Glute and hamstring, ensure you push through with your left heel, then extend your hips and draw your right knee into a hug to return to your starting position. Repeat, ensure that you complete the same number of reps on both sides.

Glute Bridge

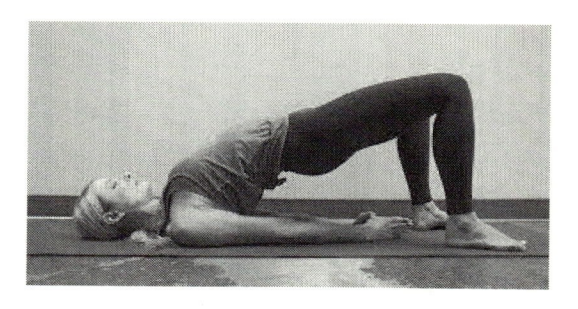

Shape.com

The Glute Bridge is an effective, versatile form of exercise that can be added to a workout routine or can be used to stretch out the glutes before you start your workout routine. This exercise can be used by anyone irrespective of age and fitness level. This exercise targets the posterior chain and the back of your legs. The posterior chain contains a group of muscles on the posterior side of a human.

Examples of the muscles on the posterior chain include the hamstring, gluteus maximus, etc. These two muscles are responsible for the bulk of the movement and strengthening these muscles will help you to increase your core stability and strengthen your lower back. There are many variations of the Glute Bridge that you can use to stretch out your glute muscles. The Glute Bridge can help to improve your posture. You do not need to have a large space to carry it out, and you do not need any extra special equipment to carry it out. You can also place a lopped resistance band above the knees to increase the intensity.

Directions

- Lie down with your face up and knees bent, and your feet planted fully on the ground pointing straight forward with little distance between both legs.
- Keep your arms at your side and your palms facing down?
- You should also ensure that your thighs are parallel to one another.
- Gently lift your hips above the ground until they are at the level of your knees, with your hips and shoulders forming a straight line.
- Doing this movement, you should ensure that your knees are over your toes during the exercise.

- Squeeze your glute muscles hard and ensure that your abs are drawn in to prevent overextension.
- Maintain this position for some seconds and then ease back down which completes one repetition.
- You should perform three sets of 15 repetitions which is also 3 rounds if you hold the position for 30 seconds.

The variations of this exercise deal with the shape and direction of the legs. You can also decide to point your legs outwards or pressing through your toes, heel, and or carrying it out on one leg. The best variation for the gluteal muscles is by pressing through the heels.

Seated hip abduction

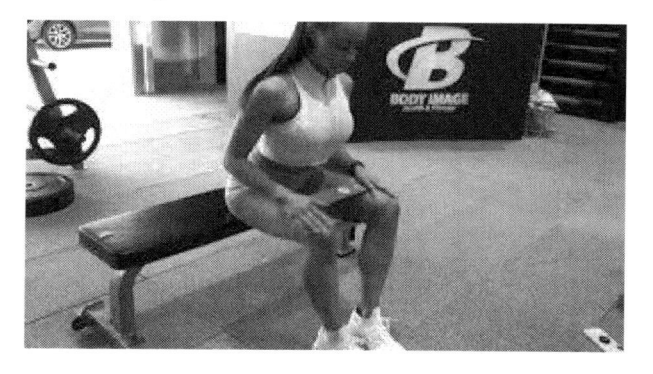

Vimeo.com

The glutes are assisted by the hip abductors to help them with some functions. These functions are standing, walking, and rotating the leg. The glutes are part of the hip abductors, and this exercise would affect them. If you are working your glutes, you should ensure that your gluteal muscles are active, and they are working to stabilize the hips.

Directions

- Put a resistance band around your lower thighs while sitting on a bench.
- Ensure that your feet on the floor are closer than the distance between the hips, although the difference should be minute.
- Lean back and place your hands on the bench you are sitting on. This position is your starting position.
- Utilize the muscles present in your glutes and hips to separate your knees and feet until they are wider than the shoulder width.

- After each movement, draw the knees back in and go back to the starting position.

Stretching Your Glutes after a Workout

Once you have completed your workout cool down for 5 minutes. After you have cooled down, you should carry out some stretches to reduce the future tightening of muscles. Here are some of the stretches that you can use to cool down or during the recovery period.

Half pigeon

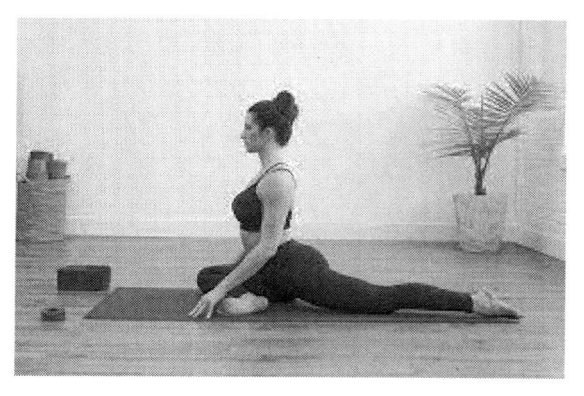

protips.dickssportinggoods.com

Directions

- Place both hands on the floor, and the distance between them should be slightly more than the normal shoulder width.
- Place both legs together, and it should be behind you and rest on the balls of your feet.
- Release your left leg, bend your knee, and put it behind you in the direction of your left wrist.
- Put your left shin in the mat, and you must make sure that your foot remains flexed.
- Simultaneously put your right knee on the mat, untuck your toes and lower your hips towards the floor.
- During this pose, ensure that you are in an upright position.
- Stay in this position for 30 seconds, five slow breaths. In this pose, it is very good to exhale as it helps sink further into your hips which benefit the stretch.
- Exhalation also helps you to maintain the level of your hips.
- Repeat this stretch with the second leg.

Standing Glute stretch

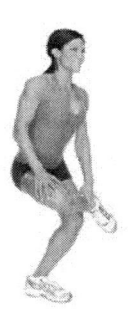

oxygenmag.com

This stretch helps to release tension as it targets the largest gluteus muscle.

Directions

- Put both feet on the floor and ensure they are shoulder-width apart.
- Lift your left leg, turn it and place the outside of your left ankle above your right knee.
- Once your left ankle is planted on your knee, bend your right knee so that you can be in a single leg squat position and push down on your left knee gently using your left elbow.

- Stay in this position for five slow breaths (30 seconds).
- Ensure that you are breathing deeply throughout the period that you are in the single-leg squat position.
- Repeat this process on the opposite side, but you should do them for the same period of time.

Some people find it hard to balance in this position. If you are one of them, there are some things that can make this process easier for you. You can focus on a spot that is close to you, or you can rest your leg on a bench or ledge that is at a hip height which would make it easier to carry out this routine. This routine can also be done while sitting with some minor changes. In the seated version, you will rest your left ankle on your right knee and lean forward with your chest.

Supine glutes stretch

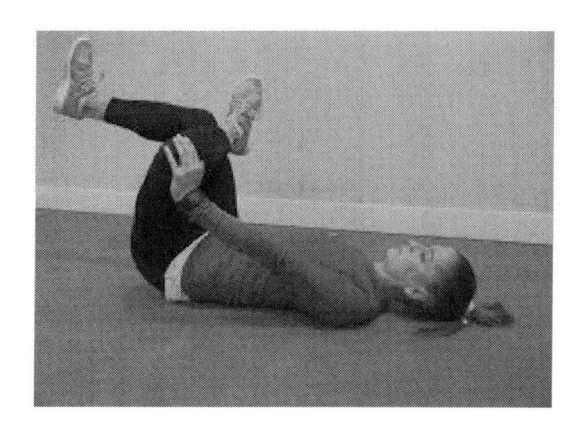

Blogpursuit.com

This stretch helps to increase the flexibility of your hip by stretching your glutes. You should use a yoga mat for this routine.

Directions

- Lie flat on your back on the yoga mat. Bend your knees and plant your feet firmly on the mat. You should ensure that the distance between your feet is hip width apart since your spine is in a neutral position.
- Lift your right leg and turn it so that the right ankle on your left leg a little above the knee.

- Pull your left knee closer to your torso by using both hands on the back of your left thigh.
- Stay in this position for 30 seconds, breathe deeply throughout this routine.
- After each exhalation, pull your knee closer to your chest.
- You can increase the stretch by pressing your right elbow into your right knee, which ensures that your spine remains in its natural position and the tailbone remains on the floor.
- You can repeat this stretch on the other side.

Static stretches

In case you were wondering, there are some glutes stretching exercises where there is little or no movement. They are called static stretches, and they are the most common and familiar type of stretching. In this stretch, you will have to hold a position for a long time, and it can be used to different types of muscles. Static exercises should only be carried out in positions where you are comfortable and can move any part of the body needed for the exercise.

There are some static stretches that can be used for glutes which will be discussed in this chapter. These exercises can be performed in a chair, and they will help you stretch out the gluteal muscles; this type of stretching is advised for people who sit at a desk for most of the day or are in a long flight or on a long car trip, and you do not like sitting on the ground. Here are some examples of glute stretches that you can do during those actions.

Seated figure-four stretches

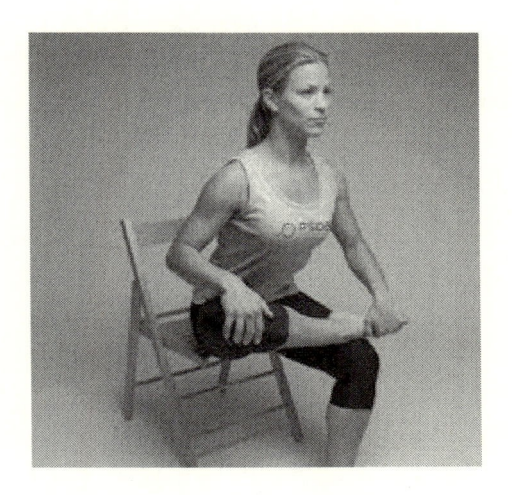

Skimble.com

This stretch is also known as the seated pigeon. You can use this stretch to loosen up your glutes and the muscles around them.

Directions

- Start by sitting upright in a solidly built chair. The next thing you should do is to rest your right ankle on your left thigh right above the knee.
- Put both hands on your shins.

- In this stretch, it is essential that your spine is straight during this exercise. With a straight spine, lean forward slightly to make the stretch deeper.
- Stay in this position for 20-30 seconds, and then go back to your initial position.
- Repeat this process with the other leg.

The static stretch can also be carried out while sitting on the ground and standing.

Seated glutes stretch

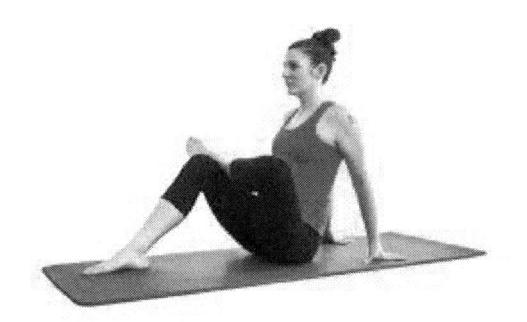

Theepochtimes.com

This is a simple stretch that would help you to relieve the tightness in your glutes, back, and hip. The way you carry out this stretch can be impacted by personal differences. For example, if you want more support for your hips, you should sit on a folded towel or on a yoga block.

Directions

- Sit on the floor or on a yoga mat and extend your legs out in front of you
- Ensure that your back is straight, keep it straight and raise your left leg and place your left ankle on your right knee.
- Make the stretch deeper by leaning slightly forward.
- Stay in this position for 20 seconds and repeat the process on the opposite side.
-

Downward-facing dog

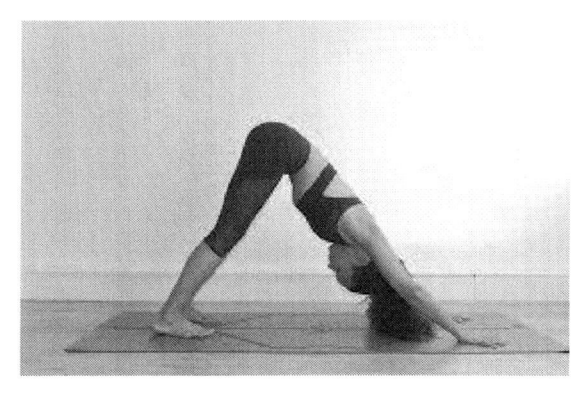

bayleafyoga.com

The downward-facing dog is a traditional yoga pose that allows you to stretch many muscles. It helps the upper body, hamstrings, glutes, and calves.

Directions

- Start by lying down in a pushup position with your hands shoulder-width apart and your legs staying together.
- Engage your core by straightening the body

- Raise your hips by moving them back and up, which should put you in an upside-down V with your body.
- Bend your knees slightly and place your head between your shoulders, and it should be in line with your spine.
- Reach your heels toward the floor but ensure that they are slightly raised
- Stay in this position for 20 seconds and then go back to your initial position.

If you want extra wrist support, you should place each hand on a yoga block. You can also bend your knees if you need it. Bending your knees would help you to straighten your back and ensure that your body remains in an upside-down V shape form.

Pigeon stretches

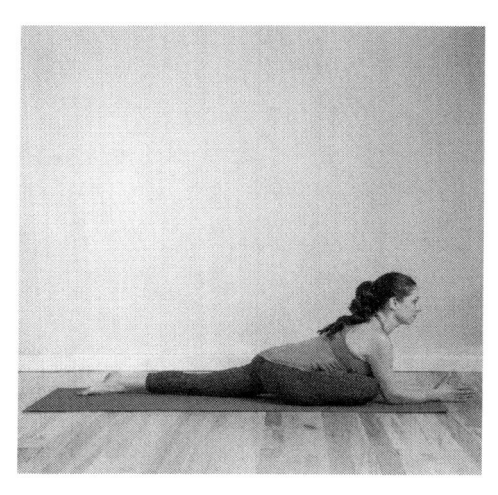

popsugar.com

This is similar to the downward-facing dog, and this stretch is commonly used in yoga. The pigeon stretch is a basic yoga move that can help you to release tension in your back, glutes, and hips.

Directions

- You should start on all fours. Lay your right knee close to your right wrist

and ensure that your shin is placed on the floor.
- Move your right ankle toward your left wrist.
- Move your left leg back, point your toes and face your hips forward.
- Extend your spine
- Proceed by moving your hands forward and stay in this position for 5 to 10 breaths.
- Move back to the initial position. Repeat this process after switching your legs.

You can add a quad stretch to this process if you want. This can be done by bending your back leg and point the upward foot, which would be held with your hand.

Knee to the opposite shoulder

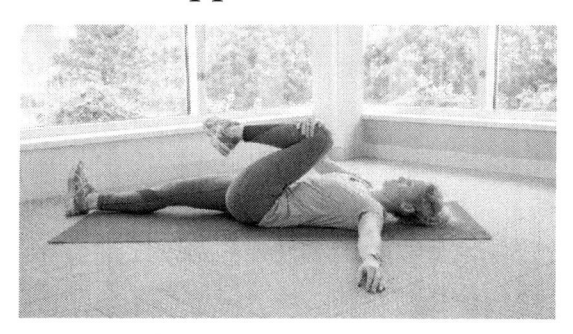

summitortho.com

This glute stretch would help people that have sciatica pain. In this static exercise, you can do it by moving your knee toward the opposite shoulder, which would help to loosen your glutes and reduce the tension around the sciatic nerve.

Directions

- Lie down on your back with legs extended and flex your feet upward
- With your hands around your knee, bend and lift your right knee.

- Move your right knee up towards your left shoulder.
- Stay in this position for 20-30 seconds, and after that, you should return your leg to the starting position.
- Repeat the process with your left leg after straightening your right leg.

In this chapter, you have learned about different stretching exercises that can work on the gluteal muscles and how you can perform them. You should know that there are different types of exercises that you can use based on your necessities.

CONCLUSION

You have just finished reading different ways that you can use to increase the size of your booty. The difference between big and small booty can be due to the accumulation of the muscles in the buttocks. There are three muscles in the gluteal region, and they are Gluteus medius, Gluteus maximus and Gluteus minimus. These muscles together are called glutes.

The shape and size of the buttocks are different between people due to our differences. The shape and size of this body part affect people differently as some start feeling insecure. You should no longer feel insecure over the size of your booty. However, we do not have total control over the development of some parts of the body. However, you can influence how your glutes will look by exercising the gluteal region's muscles. In this book, I have given you trusted exercises and stretches to use and get visible results in under thirty days. You should not only read this book but also practice and utilize it. The power to grow your glutes is now in your hand to do with it as you please. Make the best decision for yourself.

Manufactured by Amazon.ca
Bolton, ON

29546659R00143